ANESTHESIA AND THE PATIENT WITH ENDOCRINE DISEASE

ANESTHESIA AND THE PATIENT WITH ENDOCRINE DISEASE

CONTEMPORARY ANESTHESIA PRACTICE

BURNELL R. BROWN, JR., EDITOR

CASEY D. BLITT & A. H. GIESECKE, ASSOCIATE EDITORS

F. A. DAVIS COMPANY / PHILADELPHIA

Printed in the United States of America

Library of Congress Cataloging in Publication Data
Main entry under title:

Anesthesia and the patient with endocrine disease.

(Contemporary anesthesia practice; 3)
Includes bibliographical references and index.
1. Anesthesia—Complications and sequelae.
2. Endocrine glands—Surgery. I. Brown, Burnell R.
II. Blitt, Casey D. III. Giesecke, Adolph Hartung,
1932– IV. Series. [DNLM: 1. Endocrine diseases.
2. Anesthesia. W1C0769ME v. 3 / WK100 A579]
RD87.3.E53A53 617'.96 80–13067
ISBN 0–8036–1264–8

PREFACE

Nowhere is the role of the anesthesiologist as physiologist and pharmacologist more apparent and required than in the management of functioning endocrinopathies. It has been several years since a compilation of the state of the art in this field was published. Diseases of the endocrine system run the gamut from the common (diabetes) to the unusual (aldosteronoma). For the more mundane problems, several outstanding authors have been solicited for each field, so that the reader can synthesize ideas into his or her own knowledge and arrive at a preferential technique. This volume is certainly not meant to be comprehensive, but we believe it follows the philosophy of *Contemporary Anesthesia Practice* in being pragmatic and helpful in day-to-day anesthetic management.

This volume, as the others in the series, is dedicated to improved safety for our patients.

Burnell R. Brown, Jr., M.D., Ph.D.

CONTRIBUTORS

Rubin Bressler, M.D.
Professor and Head
Department of Internal Medicine
Professor
Department of Pharmacology
University of Arizona Health Sciences Center
Tucson, Arizona

Burnell R. Brown, Jr., M.D., Ph.D.
Professor and Head
Department of Anesthesiology
Professor
Department of Pharmacology
University of Arizona Health Sciences Center
Tucson, Arizona

Cecil H. Coggins, M.D.
Assistant Professor of Medicine
Harvard Medical School
Acting Chief, Renal Unit
Massachusetts General Hospital
Boston, Massachusetts

John H. Finley, M.D.
Instructor
Department of Anesthesiology
University of Arizona Health Sciences Center
Tucson, Arizona

Ronald A. Gabel, M.D.
Assistant Professor of Anesthesia
Harvard Medical School
Clinical Director and Senior Associate in Anesthesiology
Peter Bent Brigham Hospital
Boston, Massachusetts

Simon Halevy, M.D.
Professor of Anesthesiology
School of Medicine
State University of New York at Stony Brook
Director of Obstetrical Anesthesiology
Nassau County Medical Center
East Meadow, New York

Dorothea E. Hellman, M.D.
Adjunct Associate Professor
Department of Internal Medicine
University of Arizona Health Sciences Center
Consulting Endocrinologist
Tucson Hospitals Medical Education Program
Tucson, Arizona

David G. Johnson, M.D.
Associate Professor
Department of Internal Medicine
Associate Professor
Department of Pharmacology
University of Arizona Health Sciences Center
Tucson, Arizona

Rosemarie Maddi, M.D.
Assistant Professor of Anesthesia
Harvard Medical School
Fellow in Respiratory Care
Peter Bent Brigham Hospital
Boston, Massachusetts

Edward D. Miller, Jr., M.D.
Associate Professor of Anesthesiology
University of Virginia
Charlottesville, Virginia

Jordan Miller, M.D.
Associate Professor
Department of Anesthesiology
UCLA Center for the Health Sciences
Los Angeles, California

T. Oyama, M.D.
Professor
Department of Anesthesia
Hirosaki University School of Medicine
Hirosaki, Aomorioken, Japan

Daniel M. Philbin, M.D.
Assistant Professor of Anesthesia
Harvard Medical School
Associate Anesthetist
Massachusetts General Hospital
Boston, Massachusetts

Linda Stehling, M.D.
Associate Professor of Anesthesiology and Pediatrics
Upstate Medical Center
State University of New York
Syracuse, New York

Steven L. Suffecool, M.D.
Research Fellow
Department of Anesthesiology
University of Arizona Health Sciences Center
Tucson, Arizona

Hugo V. Villar, M.D.
Associate Professor
Department of Surgery
University of Arizona Health Sciences Center
Tucson, Arizona

Leonard F. Walts, M.D.
Professor
Department of Anesthesiology
UCLA Center for the Health Sciences
Los Angeles, California

Stephen L. Wangensteen, M.D.
Professor and Head
Department of Surgery
University of Arizona Health Sciences Center
Tucson, Arizona

CONTENTS

III

ANESTHETIC CONSIDERATIONS FOR ADRENALECTOMY

Rosemarie Maddi, M.D. and
Ronald A. Gabel, M.D.

Drs. Maddi and Gabel describe the anesthetic management of patients for adrenalectomy as practiced at the Peter Bent Brigham Hospital in Boston. They succinctly outline their formula for steroid replacement during such surgery and describe monitoring techniques, positioning, and other fundamentals associated with this type of endocrine surgery.

Burnell R. Brown, Jr.

Gram for gram, there is probably no tissue in the human body whose functional or structural abnormalities present more of a challenge to the anesthetist than the adrenal glands. This chapter will deal with the anesthetic considerations for adrenalectomy to extirpate the adrenal cortex, while another will deal with disorders of the adrenal medulla.

ANATOMY AND PHYSIOLOGY OF THE ADRENAL GLANDS

The adrenal glands, each weighing 3 to 6 gm, lie retroperitoneally as flattened pyramidal caps on the kidneys. Their rich blood supply, normally 6 to 7 ml/gm/min, derives from one or more inferior phrenic arteries above, from the renal arteries below, and from the aorta medially. A short central vein of the right adrenal drains directly into the vena cava, while on the left a longer common vein usually extends downward to the renal vein. Smaller venous channels also connect to the vena cava and to the splanchnic, splenic, and pancreatic veins, directing some effluent blood to the portal circulation.[1]

Two embryologically distinct layers of the adrenal gland, the cortex and the medulla, are functionally and structurally unique. The medulla, of ectodermal origin, develops from primitive cells of the sympathetic nervous system, while the cortex is derived from mesothelial buds that project bilaterally into the celom at the root of the dorsal mesentery.[1]

Major hormones secreted by the adrenal cortex are cortisol, a glucocorticoid whose primary function is the control of carbohydrate, protein, and fat metabolism; and aldosterone, a mineralocorticoid involved in the control of electrolyte metabolism. Excessive amounts of circulating cortisol lead to extensive functional and structural changes: impaired wound healing, interference with the maintenance of strong bones, lysis of lymphoid tissue, weakening of connective tissue, suppression of the inflammatory response, and reduction of the threshhold for electrical excitation of the brain, leading to psychiatric disturbances.[1]

Elevated levels of aldosterone cause a reduction in the concentration of potassium in both blood and tissue, which can produce hypochloremic alkalosis, as well as severe abnormalities in cardiac and neuromuscular function. Hypokalemia leads to electrocardiographic patterns involving combinations of flattened T waves, prominent U waves, prolongation of the QT and PR intervals, and depression of ST segments. Bradycardia and ventricular arrhythmias, including ventricular fibrillation, can result from hypokalemia. Weakness of skeletal muscles, sometimes including the diaphragm, is seen when tissue potassium levels become abnormally low.[1, 6]

Cortisol, strongly bound to protein, has a half-life in plasma of 80 to 100 minutes and is largely metabolized by the liver. Aldosterone, also hepatically reduced, has a more rapid metabolic turnover owing to weak protein binding.[1]

In addition to glucocorticoids and mineralocorticoids, the adrenal cortex also secretes steroids with estrogenic and androgenic potential. If not formulated directly in the adrenals, testosterone and estrogens are peripherally conjugated, probably in the liver, from steroids of adrenal origin.[1] Therefore, functioning tumors of the adrenal cortex can cause virilization in women and feminization in men. Furthermore, adrenalectomy is sometimes performed, along with oophorectomy or orchiectomy, to reduce levels of circulating estrogens or testosterone for the palliative treatment of metastatic cancer of the breast or prostate, respectively.

ADRENAL SURGERY

The first adrenocortical tumor may have been excised as early as 1899, and a substantial experience in adrenal surgery was gained over the next 30 years. By 1940, the adrenocortical steroids had been isolated, identified, and synthesized, which permitted the first long-term survival of a patient having bilateral total adrenalectomy in 1951.[3]

The major indications for adrenal surgery are tumors of the adrenal cortex, adrenal hyperplasia, and metastatic carcinoma of the breast. Adrenocortical tumors, usually adenoma or carcinoma, may or may not lead to excessive hormonal secretions. Signs of hypersecretion include Cushing's syndrome, virilism in women, feminism in men, and the syndrome of hypertension, hypokalemia, and vasopressin-resistant polyuria associated with primary hyperaldosteronism.[1, 3]

Adrenocortical tumors are the cause of Cushing's syndrome about 20 percent of the time, and of these, about half are benign adenomas, about half carcinomas. Bilateral adrenal hyperplasia without pituitary tumor accounts for another 25 percent, leaving ACTH-secreting tumors to account for the remainder. Forty percent of patients with Cushing's syndrome have a secreting pituitary tumor, while 15 percent have excessive ACTH originating from ectopic tissues such as the testis, prostate, parotid gland, pancreas, or an oat-cell tumor of the lung. Whereas pituitary Cushing's syndrome is three to five times as common in women as in men, the ectopic variety is largely a disease of men.[1, 2]

The adrenogenital syndrome in both men and women can be caused by adrenocortical hyperplasia or tumor, although tumors are the more common cause, and they are usually malignant. Feminizing adrenal tumors in men are typically large and highly malignant, often with both local (kidney and pancreas) and distant metastases (liver and lungs).[3]

Adrenocortical carcinomas leading to hyperfunctional disorders are characterized by autonomy such that the administration of dexamethasone fails to suppress and ACTH fails to stimulate steroid secretion by the tumor. Although the function of an adenoma is not always suppressed by dexamethasone, it can usually be stimulated by ACTH.[1, 3]

Hyperaldosteronism usually results from bilateral adrenal hyperplasia or from small adenomas, sometimes multiple, occasionally bilateral. This problem is about twice as common in women as in men. Rarely are aldosterone-secreting tumors malignant. In contrast, nonfunctioning tumors of the adrenal gland are usually malignant and are often not diagnosed before they become large abdominal masses or have metastasized to the lungs or liver. Nonfunctioning adrenal carcinoma is more common in men than in women.[1, 3]

Finally, bilateral adrenalectomy, following or simultaneous with bilateral oophorectomy or orchiectomy, is a useful palliative therapy for metastatic carcinoma of the breast or prostate. The rationale for this is that metastases from these organs tend to be metabolically dependent upon the same hormones as the parent tissues. Therefore, mammary or prostatic metastases may atrophy or involute when deprived of estrogens or androgens, respectively.

Preanesthetic Assessment

In addition to a thorough evaluation of the patient's general medical condition and anesthetic history, common to all preanesthetic visits, a few specific points related to the patient's adrenal or metastatic disease are of particular importance. In the case of an adrenocortical tumor, the anesthetist should try to ascertain the estimated size and degree of vascularity of the tumor and whether or not there is likely to be locally invasive metastases that would make adrenalectomy difficult and bloody. Review of angiograms often provides valuable information. The surgeon should be consulted to find out how the patient will be positioned on the operating table, as well as whether the operation is expected to be unilateral or is to involve bilateral exploration.

When adrenal surgery is being performed for primary hyperaldosteronism, it is essential to review the serum electrolytes and the degree of control of hypertension. In most instances, aldosterone antagonists and supplemental potassium will have been given, and sodium withheld, to correct the hypokalemia and to help bring down the blood pressure. If, however, the serum potassium remains below normal units, the anesthetist should recommend that elective adrenal surgery be postponed until further potassium therapy is administered, because of the acknowledged increased anesthetic risks engendered by hypokalemia.[6]

In addition to assessing serum electrolytes and the blood pressure of patients with Cushing's syndrome, radiographs of the bones should be reviewed for evidence of severe osteoporosis and for subclinical pathological fractures. Likewise, the metastatic bone survey of patients with metastatic mammary or prostatic cancer should be reviewed, in order to make every effort to avoid pathologic fracture of weakened bones when positioning the patient on the operating table after induction of anesthesia for adrenalectomy.

Where adrenalectomy is a palliative treatment for an inoperable nonpituitary ACTH-secreting tumor (oat-cell carcinoma, bronchial or intestinal carcinoid, islet-cell carcinoma), the patient should be evaluated for hypersecretion of other endocrine substances, such as serotonin.

Anesthetic Management

ANESTHETIC AGENTS

There are no cogent reasons to choose one over another of the available anesthetic agents or methods. Halothane, enflurane, or a balanced technique, including an appropriate neuromuscular blocker, can be selected according to the personal preference of the anesthetist.

MONITORING

The decision regarding monitoring of the patient's physiologic status during adrenal surgery depends upon the preanesthetic assessment of the patient's condition and the anticipated magnitude of surgical trauma and blood loss. If a poor-risk patient with multiple medical problems has a malignant adrenal tumor that is massive, highly vascular, and locally invasive, monitoring should probably include radial and pulmonary artery pressures; intermittent arterial blood Po_2, Pco_2, pH, and hematocrit; urine output; heart and breath sounds by esophageal stethoscope; electrocardiograph; esophageal or rectal temperature; and evaluation of the state of neuromuscular blockade by intermittent nerve stimulation. At least two short 14- or 16-gauge plastic intravenous cannulas would be essential, along with facility to warm blood to body temperature before administration. There may be some benefit from the microfiltration of blood when large volumes are infused. Six to eight units of whole blood or packed cells should be available, along with large amounts of lactated Ringer's solution.

At the other extreme, an otherwise healthy young person with mild Cushing's syndrome, having diagnostic studies suggestive of a small adrenocortical adenoma, could probably adequately be monitored by esophageal stethoscope, blood pressure cuff, electrocardiograph, temperature thermister, and nerve stimulator. One 16-gauge intravenous cannula would be sufficient, as would availability of two to four units of bank blood.

PATIENT POSITION

Position of the patient undergoing adrenal surgery is chosen according to the specifics of a given case. For example, when bilateral adrenalectomy is carried out for adrenocortical hyperplasia in the absence of an ACTH-secreting tumor, the adrenal glands are usually approached through posterolateral incisions with the patient in the lateral decubitus position, thus permitting retroperitoneal exposure in obese Cushingoid patients; the patient is turned from side to side to expose the second adrenal. In contrast, excision of normal adrenals when palliating metastatic mammary or prostatic carcinoma is commonly performed through bilateral posterior incisions, with the patient prone. For the removal of large adrenal tumors, the patient is usually positioned in the lateral decubitus position, the flank incision often involving resection of the twelfth and sometimes the eleventh rib. For massive adrenal tumors, a thoracoabdominal approach may be required to give adequate exposure.

The usual precautions of protecting the eyes from abrasion, peripheral nerves from stretch or pressure, and bony prominences from pressure should be observed. Details of positioning patients for adrenal surgery can be reviewed in Imrie and Moffitt[4] and Smith.[5] Additionally, in the patient with osteoporosis or metastatic bone disease, extreme care should be exercised in moving and positioning the patient so that brittle bones are not fractured.

PULMONARY VENTILATION

Controlled ventilation is especially desirable for adrenal surgery, even in the absence of a thoracoabdominal incision, because of the proximity of the adrenal glands to the pleura. Because pneumothorax is a common complication of adrenal surgery, the anesthetist should carefully auscult before the incision is closed to ascertain whether or not this complication has occurred. Intrapleural air can easily be removed by closure of the pleural defect with a purse-string suture over a small catheter; the air is expelled by a few large positive pressure inflations of the lungs just before the catheter is withdrawn and the suture tied.

STEROID MANAGEMENT

Supplemental steroids are usually administered during the perioperative period. This applies to patients undergoing unilateral as well as those requiring bilateral adrenalectomy, especially if the tumorous adrenal is hypersecreting, because the contralateral adrenal may well be quiescent owing to a low level of ACTH.

Some, however, do not think it necessary to administer supplemental steroids to patients undergoing unilateral adrenalectomy for aldosteronoma.

A typical steroid regimen involves the intramuscular injection of cortisone acetate (50–100 mg) on the morning of surgery, followed by the intravenous infusion of 100 mg hydrocortisone during the surgery and an additional 200 mg intravenous hydrocortisone during the remainder of the day of surgery. Daily doses are thereafter tapered over 5 days or so, from 300 to 75 mg hydrocortisone if intravenous therapy is used, or from 100 to 25 mg t.i.d. cortisone acetate if intramuscular or oral administration is chosen. Maintenance steroid replacement following bilateral adrenalectomy is usually 25 mg cortisone acetate by mouth twice a day.

Mineralocorticoids are usually given in conjunction with cortisone acetate in a dose of 0.1 mg of 9-alpha fluorohydrocortisone every other day. If patients have edema, hypertension, hypokalemia, or effusions, it is withheld. Rare patients with postural hypotension may require daily 9-alpha fluorohydrocortisone for relief.

Postanesthetic Follow-Up

As always, it is good practice for the anesthetist to evaluate the patient during the postoperative period for general medical and surgical interest, as well as for evidence of anesthetic complications. A chest radiograph in the immediate postoperative period is probably indicated to rule out pneumothorax. Additionally, the patient's postoperative fluid and electrolyte status should be followed closely, along with assessment for pathologic fractures or other complications of positioning for adrenalectomy.

ACKNOWLEDGMENTS

The authors would like to express sincere thanks to J. Hartwell Harrison, M.D., and Richard E. Wilson, M.D., surgeons having extensive experience with adrenalectomy, for their helpful suggestions.

REFERENCES

1. Dluhy, R. G., Gittes, R. F., and Harrison, J. H.: "The Adrenals." In Harrison, J. H., Gittes, R. F., Perlmutter, A. D., et al. (eds.): *Campbell's Urology.* ed. 4. W. B. Saunders, Philadelphia, 1979, pp. 2559–2640.
2. Gold, E. M.: *The Cushing syndromes: changing views of diagnosis and treatment.* Ann. Int. Med. 90:829–844, 1979.
3. Harrison, J. H., Mahoney, E. M., and Bennett, A. H.: *Tumors of the adrenal cortex.* Cancer 32:1227–1235, 1973.
4. Imrie, D. D., and Moffitt, E. A.: "The lateral decubitus position. Anesthesiologic considerations." In Martin, J. T. (ed.): *Positioning in Anesthesia and Surgery.* W. B. Saunders, Philadelphia, 1978, pp. 124–141.
5. Smith, R. H.: "The prone position." In Martin, J. H. (ed.): *Positioning in Anesthesia and Surgery.* W. B. Saunders, Philadelphia, 1978, pp. 32–43.
6. Vaughan, R. S., and Lunn, J. N.: *Potassium and the anesthetist. A review.* Anaesthesia 28:118–131, 1973.

2

ANESTHETIC MANAGEMENT FOR INSULINOMA RESECTION

Steven L. Suffecool, M.D.

Insulinoma excision is certainly not an everyday career experience for most anesthesiologists. The major concern is prevention of brain damage caused by hypoglycemia. Because of this concern, the classic method of managing these cases has been to maintain rampant hyperglycemia throughout the operative period. This concept is now being challenged. Dr. Suffecool describes an alternate technique, which is 180 degrees out of phase with the hyperglycemic maintenance protocol. CNS symptoms of hypoglycemia occur at glucose levels of 30 to 40 mg/100 ml. The majority of patients with insulinoma have had glucose levels drawn during attacks and their threshold symptomatic level has been documented. With this information, their glucose levels can be maintained above symptomatic CNS levels, but in a hypoglycemic range. The advantage of this is that excision of the insulinoma can be immediately judged adequate therapeutically by a prompt (usually 10–15 minutes) rise in glucose. The relative merits of this management versus the classic hyperglycemic technique need to be compared. Certainly there are cogent advantages, although a narrow line needs to be walked, for the system described and advocated by Dr. Suffecool.

Burnell R. Brown, Jr.

Insulinoma is a functioning endocrine tumor derived from the beta cell of the pancreatic islets of Langerhans. The tumor releases insulin and presents clinically with sequelae of hypoglycemia. Surgical resection is the only curative procedure. The responsibilities of the anesthesiologist are dual. Most important is protection of the patient from brain damage secondary to hypoglycemia. The anesthesiologist may also be instrumental in designing and conducting a perioperative plan of care that can yield important information regarding the adequacy of pancreatic resection. Topics included in this discussion are the clinical presentation of the disease, its pathophysiology, guidelines to perioperative evaluation and care of the patient, and suggested plans of anesthetic management.

Ninety percent of functioning islet cell tumors are benign adenomas referred to as insulinomas. They may become clinically significant at any age but are commonly diagnosed between the ages of 30 and 60. Episodes of hypoglycemia increase in frequency and severity insidiously, which may delay diagnosis and surgical treatment. Severe hypoglycemic states result in the typical picture of excess epinephrine levels with tremulousness, tachycardia, palpitations, and diaphoresis. Usually symptoms are limited to those caused by lack of cerebral glucose. Patients exhibit altered mental states, which may progress from mild affective disorders and confusion to frank psychosis, generalized seizure, and irreversible central nervous system damage with death. Symptomatic periods occur after prolonged fasting and may be exacerbated by alcohol. Many patients control symptoms by frequent meals. A significant portion of these patients are obese. A positive familial history of insulinoma should alert the clinician to investigate for other endocrine abnormalities. In these cases of familial multiple endocrine adenomatosis, insulinoma can be associated with other functioning endocrine tumors of the pituitary, adrenal, thyroid, and parathyroid glands (Sipple's syndrome). In these rare individuals, careful evaluation must be performed to exclude the existence of other functioning tumors such as pheochromocytoma and parathyroid adenoma.[5]

The classic triad of Whipple is valid in diagnosis of the tumor. Its elements are: (1) signs and symptoms of hypoglycemia, (2) serum blood glucose of less than 50 d/L during a symptomatic period, and (3) relief of symptoms following administration of glucose. Radioimmunoassay techniques now allow correlation of serum insulin levels with glucose concentrations verifying inappropriate insulin release. Localization of the tumor may be accomplished in approximately 60 percent of cases by celiac angiography. Clinically apparent adenomas may be as small as 15 mm in diameter, but are usually 3 to 6 cm in size. They may be found in any portion of the pancreas in ectopic locations, most commonly in the duodenum. Multiple functioning adenomas may exist. These might not be detected by preoperative angiography or even by gross inspection at the time of pancreatic resection.

Preoperative preparation of the patient for resection of insulinoma is best performed in cooperation with the surgeon and clinical pathologist. History and physical examination should document all residual neurologic damage secondary to previous hypoglycemic states. This includes assessment of cerebral function and peripheral nervous system status. When possible the level of serum glucose at which symptoms occur should be determined from chart review. If the radial artery is to be cannulated, adequate ulnar collateral flow should be documented. The patient should be aware of the risks of hypoglycemia during anesthesia and of the possibility of neurologic damage. The obese patient is prepared for the possibility of postoperative ventilatory assistance. An intravenous cannula is established when the patient is admitted to the hospital and all medications used to decrease insulin release are discontinued (diazoxide). The intravenous line allows infusion of glucose as necessary. The patient is ordered NPO after midnight. The obese patient may benefit from premedication with oral antacid. The decision to infuse dextrose-containing solutions the evening prior to surgery is predicated upon the technique of anesthetic management chosen. This is discussed in detail subsequently. Arrangements are made with the clinical pathology laboratory in advance to allow priority to be granted intraoperative blood specimens for glucose determination. This consultation must stress the necessity of rapid return of results. The clinical pathologist should be made aware that hypoglycemia may occur during operative procedure. The glucose assays commonly used in autoanalyzers may give falsely elevated results in azotemic sera. This could result in mistaken acceptance of dangerously low serum glucose. If the patient is azotemic, an assay yielding more accurate results (glucose oxidase) should be substituted. Plans are also made to allow rapid transport of the samples from the operating room to the laboratory.

General anesthesia is mandated by the extensive upper abdominal dissection, which requires good muscular relaxation and controlled ventilation. The specific technique chosen can vary with individual patient requirements, but a rational management plan is based upon the use of anesthetic drugs to decrease the cerebral demand for its major metabolic substrate, glucose. Many in vitro animal and human studies have demonstrated that several anesthetic agents decrease the cerebral metabolic rate as reflected by the consumption of oxygen by the brain ($CMRO_2$). Because glucose is the primary metabolic substrate for cerebral respiration, it has been postulated that decrease in oxygen consumption reflects a decrease in the cerebral metabolism of glucose. In vivo and animal investigations have shown in the presence of certain anesthetics that a gradual increase in brain glycogen content and high energy phosphates occurs. The protection of the human brain from hypoglycemia by anesthetic drugs cannot be demonstrated directly for obvious ethical reasons. The information concerning mammalian brain does suggest that use of an agent that decreases $CMRO_2$ is a rational choice when concern about hypoglycemia exists.[2, 6, 7]

Enflurane is a potent attenuator of $CMRO_2$. It has been reported to decrease oxygen consumption 50 percent when inspired concentration is 3 percent.[9] Halothane also significantly decreases $CMRO_2$, but has been observed to increase sensitivity to insulin in the periphery. This may be important if patients are to be managed with moderate hypoglycemia. Halothane may also not be the agent of first choice because of the probability of hepatobiliary diversion being performed for adequate exposure. The risk of postoperative obstructive jaundice is significant and diagnosis could be obscured. Barbiturate and neuroleptic techniques result in a significant decrease in $CMRO_2$, but require high concentrations of inspired nitrous oxide. The ability to deliver high inspired oxygen concentrations may become important in ventilating patients undergoing prolonged retroperitoneal dissection. As mentioned earlier, a significant portion of the patients are obese, which may further complicate intraoperative respiratory care.

The induction of anesthesia can be safely accomplished with

thiopental unless otherwise contraindicated. Ketamine should be avoided because of its capacity for increasing $CMRO_2$. Controlled mechanical ventilation is instituted with minute ventilation adequate to maintain normocarbia. Hypocarbia should be avoided because of the decrease in cerebral blood flow and consequent decrease in glucose delivery.

As mentioned previously the intraoperative maintenance of adequate levels of serum glucose is of paramount importance. Logistical problems concerning rapid determinations of serum glucose are clarified prior to the date of surgery. A convenient access for blood samples is established prior to the induction of anesthesia. An intraarterial cannula is useful for this and also allows the anesthesiologist rapid analysis of perfusion pressure and respiratory status. The maintenance of serum glucose is approached in one of two ways. Classically an excess amount of serum glucose is administered to eliminate any possibility of intraoperative hypoglycemia.[1, 3, 4] An infusion of dextrose (5 or 10 percent) is begun the evening prior to the operation and continued through the procedure. Ten percent dextrose has been preferred by some physicians because of the theoretical risk of release of large amounts of insulin during manipulation of the tumor. This risk has not been substantiated, and in the few cases in which insulin levels have been correlated to tumor manipulation the levels of circulating insulin have not increased significantly.[8] Plasma glucose should be monitored frequently during the case. Samples should be tested immediately prior to the induction of anesthesia and at least every 30 minutes thereafter, including in the recovery room. These latter samples are of great importance for two reasons. First, the patient is at risk for rebound hyperglycemia following resection of the tumor. Second, there may exist multiple adenomas that were not apparent during resection, and these could result in hypoglycemia during the early postoperative period.

The second method of glucose manipulation has the patient moderately hypoglycemic throughout the operation. The reason for this management is to allow rapid assessemnt of the adequacy of pancreatic resection. If the entire insulin-secreting mass is removed, one expects to see a rapid increase in serum glucose levels. This information can be correlated with previous angiographic evidence and gross anatomic inspection to determine whether further resection is necessary. A rise in the serum glucose after removal of the mass is suggestive of adequate resection.[8]

The use of this technique requires meticulous monitoring of serum glucose. The night prior to surgery the patient receives infusion of solutions not containing glucose. Frequent serum glucose determinations are obtained (every 1 to 2 hours), including a sample just prior to transport to the operating room. Intermittent infusions of dextrose are employed to obviate subjective symptoms and to maintain serum glucose at approximately 50 mg percent. It is helpful to know the approximate level of serum glucose at which the individual patient becomes symptomatic. This may serve as a crude gauge for the absolute minimum serum glucose levels to be tolerated. During the course of surgery serum glucose levels are obtained every 15 minutes. It is useful to correlate these determinations with Dextrostix testing. This rapid method of serum glucose determination can be useful if it becomes necessary to infuse glucose in small amounts to regain acceptable serum levels. Following removal of the insulinoma, a rise in the serum glucose to normal fasting levels occurs in 30 to 45 minutes. This information, along with frozen section pathologic evaluation of the tissue specimen and gross exploration, suggests adequate resection. Failure of the expected rise to occur may indicate further resection is necessary. At the termination of the procedure the patient should be maintained on supplemental oxygen until alert, and glucose determinations continued until serum glucose levels stabilize.

The anesthetic management of the patient with insulinoma presents certain unique challenges, which are effectively conquered with careful preparation and rational application of appropriate anesthetic drugs. The ever present risk of hypoglycemia during the anesthesia can be minimized by vigilant monitoring of serum glucose levels. This requires a coordinated effort among the anesthesiologist, clinical pathologist, and surgeon. A plan of care using moderate levels of hypoglycemia during the operation can be used to aid in assessment of adequate pancreatic resection. A rise of serum glucose to normal fasting levels after the excision of the mass may be presumptive evidence of adequacy of pancreatectomy and spare the patient the increased morbidity associated with further resection. The general anesthetic chosen for the individual patient should be examined for its theoretical ability to protect the brain from hypoglycemia by the reduction of cerebral metabolic rate. Thiopental induction followed by enflurane maintenance with controlled ventilation with normocarbia seems a reasonable management plan. The use of the volatile agent allows high inspired oxygen concentrations to be used. This may be important in patients having prolonged high retroperitoneal dissection and compromised respiratory mechanics. A significant portion of the patients are obese, which may further increase the need for high inspired oxygen concentrations. The patient requires close observation in the postoperative period to guard against rebound hyperglycemia and hypoglycemia. The latter may be secondary to undetected multiple insulinomas.

REFERENCES

1. Bourke, A. M.: *Anaesthesia for the surgical treatment of insulinomas.* Anaesthesia 21:239–243, 1966.
2. Brunner, E. A., Passonneau, J. V., and Molstead, C.: *The effect of volatile anaesthetics on levels of metabolites and on metabolic rate in brain.* Neurochem. 18:2301–2316, 1971.
3. Colella, J. J., and Vandam, L. D.: *Diethyl ether anesthesia for a patient with hyperinsulinism.* Anesthesiology 37:354–356, 1972.
4. Fraser, R. A.: *Hyperinsulinism under anesthesia.* Anaesthesia 18:3–8, 1963.
5. Higgins, G. A.: *Endocrine surgery.* Surg. Clin. North Am. Feb.: 131–143, 1979.
6. Mayman, C. I., Gatfield, P. D., and Brecjenridge, B. M.: *The glucose content of brain in anaesthesia.* J. Neurochem. 11:483–487, 1964.
7. Nilsson, L., and Siejo, B. K.: *Influence of anaesthetics on the balance between production and utilization of energy in the brain.* J. Neurochem. 23:29–36, 1974.
8. Schnelle, N., Molnar, G. D., Ferris, D. O., et al.: *Circulating glucose and insulin in surgery for insulinomas.* J.A.M.A. 217:1072–1078, 1971.
9. Smith, A. L., and Wollman, H.: *Cerebral blood flow and metabolism: effects of anesthetic drugs and techniques.* Anesthesiology 36:378–400, 1972.

3

THE RENIN-ANGIOTENSIN SYSTEM IN ANESTHESIA

Edward D. Miller, Jr., M.D.

The renin-angiotensin system is described by Dr. Miller and the implications of this neurohumoral system for anesthesia are discussed.

Burnell R. Brown, Jr.

In 1934 Goldblatt showed that a sustained rise in arterial blood pressure could result if the renal artery of a dog was constricted.[5] Renin was demonstrated to be released from the kidney by Kohlstaedt and Page in 1940.[10] Since that time, thousands of articles examining the renin-angiotensin system in health and disease have been published. These studies suggest that renin and the subsequent conversion to angiotensin II plays an important role in blood pressure regulation and ultimately in control of body fluids. This brief review is intended to examine some of the basic information about the renin-angiotensin system, how the renin-angiotensin system is effected by anesthesia and surgery, and then finally what implications this has for anesthesiologists.

RENIN CASCADE

Renin is a highly specific proteolytic enzyme released from the kidney under a variety of stimuli. Once into the circulation, renin cleaves its substrate, an alpha-2-globulin synthesized by the liver, to produce the decapeptide (10 amino acids) angiotensin I. The decapeptide passes through the pulmonary circulation where an enzyme called *converting enzyme* clips off two amino acids to produce the octapeptide angiotensin II. The function of angiotensin I is unknown. Angiotensin II has been more extensively studied and its actions include intense vasoconstriction, positive inotropic effect on the heart, elevation of blood pressure with central administration, stimulation of drinking behavior, stimulation and potentiation of catecholamine release, and the primary stimulus to aldosterone production. Angiotensin II is thought to be broken down rapidly into inactive fragments. This was the classic view until recent work by Goodfriend and Peach, which showed that a seven amino acid unit, called angiotensin III, could be produced by the action of endogenous enzymes.[6] Angiotensin III in much smaller quantities than angiotensin II can also induce aldosterone production. Catecholamine biosynthesis is accelerated by angiotensin III through the activation of tyrosine hydroxylase, which may involve increased concentrations of either calcium or cyclic adenosine monophosphate (AMP). Prostaglandin synthesis is also induced by angiotensin III as well as angiotensin II. It would appear that several peptide fragments other than angiotensin II have important regulatory roles.

One reason for the slow advance in the field has been the inability to measure renin easily. The early assays employed the injection of blood extracts into rats and measured an increased blood pressure. These assays were cumbersome, slow, and of uncertain specificity. During the 1960s, methods were worked out to determine renin by radioimmunoassay. Blood for analysis is taken in a chilled container to prevent enzyme breakdown. The plasma is separated and incubated in such a manner as to generate angiotensin I, which is then radioimmunoassayed. Renin activity is then reported as nanograms of angiotensin I generated per milliliter of plasma per hour of generation.[7] It should be pointed out that this assay does not measure the circulating amount of angiotensin II. It is assumed that almost complete conversion of angiotensin I to angiotensin II will occur, however.

RENIN RELEASE

Renin is released into the circulation under a variety of stimuli. There are three generally accepted mechanisms regulating the secretion of renin from the juxtaglomerular apparatus in the kidney. The first mechanism is a baroreceptor or stretch mechanism, whereby decreased pressure within the afferent arteriole of the glomerulus results in renin release. The second mechanism depends on the sodium content of the urine delivered to the distal tubule and sensed in the macula densa. The third mechanism is neurogenic in nature and depends on the rich sympathetic nerves supplying the juxtaglomerular apparatus. Increased circulating levels of vasopressin and angiotensin II depress renin secretion, whereas circulating catecholamines stimulate renin release. Any or all of these mechanisms may be involved in renin release. The anesthetic and surgical experience alters blood pressure, sympathetic nervous system activity, and kidney function, and therefore alterations in renin release are expected.

ANESTHESIA AND SURGERY

Since the release of renin is under a variety of stimuli that may be influenced by anesthetic agents, it is not surprising that plasma renin activity has been measured in several clinical settings. Robertson and Michelakis in examining 31 surgical patients found that plasma renin activity did not rise with halothane anesthesia, but once surgery had begun, plasma renin activity did rise.[18]

Pettinger and coworkers examined a series of anesthetic agents in the rat and found large increases in plasma renin activity.[16] Further work by Tanaka and Pettinger suggested that the blood pressure rise induced by ketamine in the rat was the result of renin release.[19] Patients anesthetized with ketamine anesthesia do not show a rise in plasma renin activity.[13]

Bailey and coworkers showed in patients with cardiac disease undergoing cardiopulmonary bypass with large-dose morphine-nitrous oxide anesthesia that plasma renin activity did not rise with anesthesia, but did rise once a surgical incision was made.[1] It was noted in that study that the highest plasma renin activity occurred at a point of maximal blood pressure rise after surgical incision. The effect of this rise is unknown but the potential for myocardial ischemia owing to increased work of the heart and coronary vasoconstriction from angiotensin II are real possibilities. Angiotensin II in the past had been used as a vasopressor, but lost popularity because of the angina pectoris some patients experienced when it was administered. Bailey also noted in this study that there was a marked increase in plasma aldosterone levels, which paralleled the increase in plasma renin activity. The effect of aldosterone on the kidney is to increase sodium reabsorption. The increased sodium reabsorption results in water retention, which helps increase circulating blood volume. The price the body pays for the increase in body sodium content is the loss of potassium. Bailey showed in this study that the potassium loss experienced by patients undergoing open heart surgery was due to renin-angiotensin-aldosterone mechanism.

From the data available, it appears that the smooth induction of general anesthesia by a variety of commonly used anesthetic agents does not result in an increase in plasma renin activity. However, once surgical trauma begins, plasma renin activity may increase.

As was stated previously, plasma renin activity may not reflect angiotensin II levels, since the assay quantitates angiotensin I generated. Studies in rat and man have now shown that anesthetic agents when used in clinical concentrations do not alter the conversion of angiotensin I to angiotensin II. Plasma renin activity during anesthesia is a reliable surrogate for estimating the amount of the potent vasopressor angiotensin II present.

What is the significance of the rise in plasma renin activity? It was theorized that the rise in plasma renin activity meant that more angiotensin II was in the circulation, which resulted in vasoconstriction. This vasoconstriction either maintained the blood pressure or elevated the blood pressure. However, a cause and effect relationship was not established.

Over the past several years, several inhibitors of the renin-angiotensin system have been developed. SQ 20,881 (Teprotide) blocks the conversion of angiotensin I to angiotensin II and was used to show that the initiation of renovascular hypertension in the dog was angiotensin II dependent. SQ 14,225 (Captopril) is an orally effective converting enzyme inhibitor that has recently been shown to be an effective antihypertensive agent.[4] Saralasin (sar-l-ala-8 angiotensin II) is a competitive inhibitor of angiotensin II and has been used in patients with coarctation of the aorta to demonstrate the degree of blood pressure support exerted by the renin-angiotensin system in these patients.[17]

We have used inhibitors of the renin-angiotensin system to quantitate the importance of the renin-angiotensin system in blood pressure support with various anesthetic agents in the rat. We found that when rats were anesthetized with halothane, enflurane, fluroxene, or ketamine, plasma renin activity did not rise. However, when saralasin was infused, mean arterial blood pressure decreased 20 torr with halothane and enflurane, but not with fluroxene or ketamine.[14] In animals in whom plasma renin activity is already elevated (salt depletion, hemorrhage, dehydration), blood pressure fell 30 torr when saralasin was infused either in the awake or in the anesthetized state.[11] These results demonstrate that the measurement of plasma renin activity does not accurately predict the degree of blood pressure support exerted by the renin-angiotensin system during anesthesia. Since these blocking agents are still experimental drugs, they have not been infused in patients during anesthesia or surgery. There is much evidence, however, to suggest that the rat model will accurately predict the response of patients to these inhibitors. Many patients who come to the operating room are volume-depleted, either because of poor intake, nasogastric suction, chronic diuretic therapy, or fever. A significant degree of blood pressure support in these patients is due to angiotensin

II. Whether this degree of vasoconstriction to various vascular beds is harmful has not been examined.

Renin release is also known to occur when controlled hypotension is employed. Sodium nitroprusside causes a release of renin in man and animal. The elevated angiotensin II levels partially antagonize the effects of sodium nitroprusside.[12] The rebound hypertension sometimes seen when sodium nitroprusside is terminated is due to the elevated angiotensin II levels. Whether the combined use of an angiotensin antagonist and sodium nitroprusside would be beneficial in patient care has not been studied.

One other time in which renin release is known to occur is during hemorrhage. Very large increases in plasma renin activity occur with hemorrhage that is not blocked by anesthetic agents. A significant degree of blood pressure support is exerted by the renin-angiotensin system during hemorrhage.[15] Whether the elevated levels of angiotensin II are beneficial for organ perfusion has been questioned; however, studies in man have not been done.

IMPLICATIONS

The information presented demonstrates that the renin-angiotensin system is a critical component in blood pressure regulation. There are two types of patients in whom this information will directly affect us as anesthesiologists: patients who have been subjected to hemorrhage and patients with hypertension.

There is mounting evidence that in hemorrhagic shock both renin and antidiuretic hormone concentrations are elevated along with transient elevations of the prostaglandins. The role of these vasoactive substances in hemorrhagic shock is an area of extensive research. Jakschik and coworkers[8, 9] have shown that during hemorrhage in the dog, renin and catecholamines are released, and by using an angiotensin II competitive inhibitor, part of the vasoconstriction seen in the kidney is reversed. Subsequent studies have shown that while both catecholamines and prostaglandins are released during hemorrhage, their levels return toward control during the phase of decompensation, whereas renin levels remain elevated. Feuerstein and coworkers have abolished the catecholamine response to hemorrhage through the use of saralasin in cats who have hemorrhaged.[3]

Errington and coworkers have carried out similar hemorrhage experiments in dogs and have shown that with blockade of the angiotensin converting enzyme, 100 percent survival could be obtained.[2] They also performed experiments on dogs with experimental diabetes insipidus and found increased survival. From these experiments, they suggest that the vasoconstriction in the gut and kidney is prevented when antidiuretic hormone (ADH) or angiotensin II are blocked and that this accounts for the increased survival. They note, however, that angiotensin II has other effects, and the interaction with catecholamines may be equally important. Angiotensin II is known to potentiate the vasoconstrictor effects of catecholamines as well as to enhance the release of catecholamines.

How anesthetic agents affect the renin-angiotensin system during various pathologic states has not been extensively studied. However, if the intense vasoconstriction seen in patients who are in shock is detrimental, then the choice of proper anesthetic agents and judicious use of angiotensin antagonists may be beneficial. The use of blocking peptides in human hemorrhagic shock has not begun. However, the almost certain mortality of the 65-year-old man with a ruptured aortic aneurysm and impending renal failure makes the use of such agents attractive. Whether or not survival can be achieved and be properly ascribed to the use of such agents will be learned only by the use of careful clinical trials.

The second critical area in which knowledge of renin-angiotensin is important is in patients with hypertension. It had been thought with the discovery of renin that hypertension was due to the release of renin. Subsequently, however, it has been found that there are many forms of hypertension.

Patients with renovascular hypertension have initial increases in plasma renin activity. However, once the disease has progressed and we see these patients in the operating room for repair of renal artery stenosis, their plasma renin activity may be normal. This is probably due to the volume expansion that occurs when angiotensin II stimulates aldosterone production. Other patients will have elevated levels of renin throughout their disease. Some investigators believe that using inhibitors of the renin-angiotensin system will be diagnostic in patients with renal artery stenosis and have used such inhibitors as a predictor of the blood pressure response these patients will experience postoperatively. The use of these inhibitors intraoperatively versus nonspecific agents like propranolol is an attractive approach to these patients. If the anesthesiologist was using a potent inhalational agent and an inhibitor, a greater degree of blood pressure fall might be seen. Such a hypothesis has not been tested.

The majority of cases of hypertension have no known cause. Renovascular, pheochromocytoma, coarctation of the aorta, and other endocrine forms of hypertension are rare. How the renin-angiotensin system interacts with the central and peripheral sympathetic nervous system is actively being investigated. The work by Gavras and coworkers deserves comment, however.[4] They found that in 12 hypertensive patients treated with a converting enzyme inhibitor, blood pressure decreased significantly in all the patients treated. There was no significant correlation between pretreatment plasma renin activity and the degree of blood pressure fall, however. This work suggests that either this particular agent has an unknown hypotensive effect or that angiotensin II works in concert with other hormones to maintain an elevated blood pressure. Once small amounts of angiotensin II are eliminated, blood pressure is able to return toward normal levels.

It is clear that through the use of blockers of the renin-angiotensin system, new information is now available on how this system helps regulate blood pressure and fluid volume. The anesthesiologist will in the very near future see patients coming to the operating room who are currently taking such blocking agents. He may find the need to administer such agents to patients in order to improve organ perfusion or to treat hypertension. He will need to know the basic pharmacology of these drugs, much as he does for the alpha and beta antagonists that we frequently use at the present time.

REFERENCES

1. Bailey, D. R., Miller, E. D. Jr., Kaplan, J. A. et al.: *The renin-angiotensin-aldosterone system during cardiac surgery with morphine-nitrous oxide anesthesia.* Anesthesiology 42:538, 1975.

2. Errington, M., Rocha, E., and Silva, M.: *On the role of vasopressin and angiotensin in the development of irreversible hemorrhagic shock.* J. Physiol. (Lond.) 242:119–141, 1974.
3. Feuerstein, G., Boonyavirog, P., Gutman, Y., et al.: *Adrenal catecholamine response to hemorrhage abolished by an angiotensin antagonist.* Eur. J. Pharmacol. 41:85–86, 1977.
4. Gavras, H., Brunner, H., Turini, G., et al.: *Antihypertensive effect of the oral angiotensin converting enzyme inhibitor SQ14,225 in man.* N. Engl. J. Med. 298:991–95, 1978.
5. Goldblatt, H., Lynch, J., Hanzal, R. F., et al.: *Studies on experimental hypertension: production of persistent elevation of systolic blood pressure by means of renal ischemia.* J. Exp. Med. 59:347–379, 1934.
6. Goodfriend, T., and Peach, M. J.: *Angiotensin III.* Circ. Res. (suppl.) 36–37:138–48, 1975.
7. Haber, E., Koerner, T., Page, L. B., et al.: *Application of a radioimmunoassay for angiotensin I to the physiologic measurements of plasma renin activity in normal human subjects.* J. Clin. Endocrinol. 29:1349–1355, 1967.
8. Jakschik, B., Marshall, G., Kourik, J., et al.: *Profile of circulating vasoactive substances in hemorrhagic shock and their pharmacologic manipulation.* J. Clin. Invest. 54:842–852, 1974.
9. Jakschik, B., McKnight, R., Marshall, G., et al.: *Renin vascular changes during hemorrhagic shock and pharmacologic modification by angiotensin and catecholamine antagonists.* Circulatory Shock 1:231–237, 1974.
10. Kohlstaedt, K. G., and Page, I. H.: *Liberation of renin by perfusion of kidneys following reduction of pulse pressure.* J. Exp. Med. 72:201–216, 1940.
11. Miller, E. D., Ackerly, J. A., and Peach, M. J.: *Blood pressure support during general anesthesia in a renin-dependent state in the rat.* Anesthesiology 48:401–408, 1978.
12. Miller, E. D., Ackerly, J. A., Vaughan, E. D., et al.: *The renin-angiotensin system during controlled hypotension with sodium nitroprusside.* Anesthesiology 47:257–262, 1977.
13. Miller, E. D., Bailey, D., Kaplan, J., et al.: *The effect of ketamine on the renin-angiotensin system.* Anesthesiology 42:503–505, 1975.
14. Miller, E. D., Longnecker, D. E., and Peach, M. J.: *The regulatory function of the renin-angiotensin system during general anesthesia.* Anesthesiology 48:399–403, 1978.
15. Miller, E. D., Longnecker, D. E., and Peach, M. J.: *Renin response to hemorrhage in awake and anesthetized rats.* Circulatory Shock, in press.
16. Pettinger, W. A., Tanaka, K., Keeton, K., et al.: *Renin release, an*

artifact of anesthesia and its complications in rats. Proc. Soc. Exp. Biol. Med. 148:625–30, 1975.
17. Ribeiro, A., and Krakoff, L.: *Angiotensin blockade in coarctation of the aorta.* N. Engl. J. Med. 295:148–150, 1976.
18. Robertson, D., and Michelakis, A.: *Effect of anesthesia and surgery on plasma renin activity in man.* J. Clin. Endocrinol. Metab. 34:831–37, 1974.
19. Tanaka, K., and Pettinger, W. A.: *Renin release and ketamine-induced cardiovascular stimulation in the rat.* J. Pharmacol. Exp. Ther. 188:229–33, 1974.

4

THE EFFECTS OF ANESTHESIA ON ANTIDIURETIC HORMONE

Daniel M. Philbin, M.D., and
Cecil H. Coggins, M.D.

An anesthesiologist and an internist, Drs. Philbin and Coggins, form a team to describe the latest information available concerning antidiuretic hormone (ADH) and its perspective in anesthesiology. There has been confusion about the relative roles of stress, surgery, and specific anesthetic pharmacology on release and activity of this hormone. The following article summarizes the available information and denotes clinical relevance.

Burnell R. Brown, Jr.

The reduction of urinary flow and electrolyte excretion, particularly of sodium, that may occur in patients subjected to anesthesia and surgery has long been recognized. Since general anesthesia and surgical interventions are considered stressful situations for the patient and since the antidiuretic hormone (ADH) in man is a "stress response" hormone, it has also long been postulated that anesthetic drugs alone, as well as surgical stimulation, were capable of stimulating release of ADH. This hypothesis was given considerable impetus by Duke in 1951, when he and his coworkers demonstrated that the presence of morphine in the hypothalamus of dogs resulted in an inhibition of diuresis and ADH release.[2]

Until recent years, prior to the advent of specific radioimmunoassays, much of the experimental evidence for an antidiuretic hormone-releasing action for anesthesia was based upon indirect evidence or supposition. Often, too, such experiments were performed in the laboratory animal. Unfortunately, data now strongly suggest that marked species differences exist. Before discussing the more recent data available, the physiology and pharmacology of ADH will be briefly reviewed.

ANTIDIURETIC HORMONE

The antidiuretic hormone in man is arginine vasopressin, a polypeptide, which has nine amino acid residues. It is considered an octapeptide because the cysteine residues at positions 1 and 6 combine to form cystine. It is believed to be formed predominantly in the supraoptic nucleus, one of two nuclei in the hypothalamoneurohypophyseal system. Following formation, ADH is transported within the axons to be stored in the posterior pituitary pending release into the systemic circulation after a suitable stimulus. It is now known that the releasing mechanism is a calcium-dependent reaction. A large number of stimuli have been postulated or demonstrated to play a role in the release of ADH, some of which are listed in Table 1. It should be readily apparent from reviewing the table that in many situations more than one stimulus may be involved, e.g., hemorrhagic shock with concomitant stress, hypotension, and decreased blood volume. Thus it may often be difficult, if not impossible, to identify and separate a discrete single stimulus as a causal factor in ADH release.

Table 1. Stimuli for Antidiuretic Hormone Release

1. Increase in plasma osmotic pressure stimulates osmoreceptors in supraoptic and paraventricular nuclei of hypothalamus.
2. Decrease in arterial blood pressure stimulates baroreceptors in carotid sinus and/or aortic arch.
3. Decrease in intrathoracic blood volume stimulates stretch receptors in left atrium.
4. Drugs—cholinergic and β-adrenergic
5. Hypoxia
6. Hypercarbia
7. Increased body temperature
8. Stress—including pain and fear

Note: Numbers 4 through 8 may have a direct effect on the hypothalamopituitary system.

Physiologic and Pharmacologic Effects

The use of the term *antidiuretic* may be misleading, since this is but one of the hormone's recognized actions. The name *vasopressin* will be used interchangeably with ADH. We will discuss some of the functions of ADH briefly.

ANTIDIURETIC ACTION

The antidiuretic action of ADH (vasopressin) is well recognized as one of its major physiologic actions. In some circumstances, it plays a major role in altering the renal excretion of solute free water in order to maintain the osmolality and volume of body fluids. It accomplishes this by increasing the reabsorption of water in the kidney primarily in the collecting ducts by making the luminal cell membranes more permeable to water. The mechanism for this action has not been clearly delineated but it is known to involve the enzymatic formation of cyclic adenosine monophosphate (AMP) in the kidney. Following its formation, the cyclic AMP can then affect water permeability in two ways: either by changes within the microfilaments or microtubles or by involvement in cyclic AMP-dependent phosphorylation of specific proteins. The relative contribution of either system remains unknown.

The net result is an increase in the water permeability of the tubules, with more water being reabsorbed, thereby leaving behind a more concentrated urine of smaller volume. An indirect measurement of this action can be calculated by determining the reduction in free water clearance that occurs:

$$C_{H2O} = V - C_{osm} \qquad C_{osm} = \frac{U_{osm} \times V}{P_{osm}}$$

where

C_{H2O} = Free water clearance
V = Urinary flow ml/min
C_{osm} = Solute clearance
U_{osm} = Urine osmolality (mOsm/kg)
P_{osm} = Plasma osmolality (mOsm/kg)

The effect then is a reduction in free water clearance and volume, without reducing solute clearance. It should be noted here that such an antidiuretic action occurs at very low concentrations of ADH and that levels beyond the range of 15 pg/ml produce no further antidiuretic action, and indeed may have a reverse effect.

VASOPRESSOR ACTION

The vasopressor action of ADH is another of its major effects that is well recognized. It is an extremely potent vasoconstrictor in man, perhaps more potent than angiotensin.[9] It has a direct effect on the smooth muscle of vascular beds and seems to have its major effect on the splanchnic, renal, and coronary beds. Such an action is the basis for the use of exogenous vasopressin preparations in the management of gastrointestinal bleeding. The coronary vascular effect may also explain the occasional fatal complication of acute myocardial infarction following its administration.

The net effect of vasopressin (ADH) is to increase peripheral vascular resistance and decrease cardiac output and stroke volume. However, it also has been noted to decrease pulmonary artery pressure, an action that has been used with some success in management of patients with pulmonary hemorrhage.[18] The levels of endogenous ADH required to produce a vasopressor effect in man are such that in the past this was not generally considered to be of any clinical significance. However, more recent data suggest that such responses may occur at levels considerably below those previously thought necessary and may, therefore, play a role in some clinical situations, e.g., stimulation during "light" anesthesia.[11]

DIURETIC-NATRIURETIC ACTION

The diuretic-natriuretic effect of ADH represents an interesting physiologic paradox. As mentioned previously, in low concentrations ADH can significantly decrease the volume and increase the concentration of urine produced by the kidney. In high concentrations, however, a reverse effect has been noted, with an increase in urine volume and a corresponding increase in urinary sodium excretion.[7] This has been reasonably well demonstrated in animal preparations, although the mechanism of action remains unclear. There is evidence to suggest that in high concentrations, vasopressin inhibits sodium reabsorption in the distal as well as the proximal kidney tubule.[6, 19] It can also alter the distribution of renal blood flow, which may in itself be a factor in urine formation.[5] Such a diuretic effect has been produced in animals even when the hypertensive effects of the vasopressin were ablated by the administration of sodium nitroprusside.

The levels of ADH required for this effect are so far beyond the range for a physiologic antidiuretic action on the kidney that it is believed to be of no clinical significance in man. However, in special circumstances, e.g., cardiopulmonary bypass, such concentrations have been reported[13, 16] and may indeed be playing a role.

EFFECT OF ANESTHETICS

As was mentioned in the introduction, oliguria and decreased urinary electrolyte excretion are frequently noted following anesthesia and operation. Much of the early work in this area focused upon a direct mechanism for the release of antidiuretic hormone by narcotics and general anesthetics. Unfortunately this approach tends to ignore a number of the actions of the anesthetics themselves, which can produce a nonADH-mediated oliguria or may lead to a secondary release of ADH. All too often such studies also failed to differentiate between the effects of anesthesia and those of the surgical stimulation. Table 2 lists some of these mechanisms.

It should be apparent that if an anesthetic such as halothane produces a decrease in both renal blood flow and glomerular

Table 2. Possible Mechanisms for Oliguria during Anesthesia and Surgery

1.	Decreased cardiac output—decreased renal blood flow
2.	Hypotension—decreased renal blood flow
3.	Impaired autoregulation of renal blood flow
4.	Altered distribution of renal blood flow
5.	Dehydration—inadequate fluid replacement
6.	Increased renal vascular resistance
7.	Alteration of renal tubular transport mechanism
8.	Stimulation of the renin-angiotensin system
9.	Release of antidiuretic hormone

filtration rate, it is not necessary to involve an ADH mechanism to explain any decrease in urine formation. In addition, there are a number of other factors, listed in the table, that can contribute to or be responsible for perioperative oliguria.

Nonetheless, the theory that anesthetics (and narcotics) result in a direct release of ADH received considerable support from these early studies. Such studies, however, used indirect evidence for an ADH effect (e.g., decrease in free water clearance) or utilized a biologic assay that was tedious, time consuming, and of limited value. The development of specific radioimmunoassays for vasopressin has led to renewed interest in this area.[10, 14] Subsequent studies utilizing such an assay have reexamined the ADH response to many of the commonly used anesthetics.

In our laboratories a series of studies using radioimmunoassays were performed in surgical patients.[11, 14] In the first of these studies patients scheduled for elective cardiac surgery were followed. Anesthesia consisted of morphine 1 mg/kg and 50 percent oxygen-50 percent nitrous oxide. Measurements made before induction of anesthesia, at 15 and 30 minutes after induction, and at 15 and 30 minutes during operation revealed no significant alteration in ADH levels during the anesthesia period alone. Following surgical incision there were marked rises in ADH. Subsequent studies with halothane and morphine 2 mg/kg confirmed these findings (Fig. 1). Similar results have been reported by other investigators with the same anesthetics.[3, 16] This seems to indicate that the ADH response attributed to anesthesia in earlier studies was really reflecting the response to surgical stimulation.

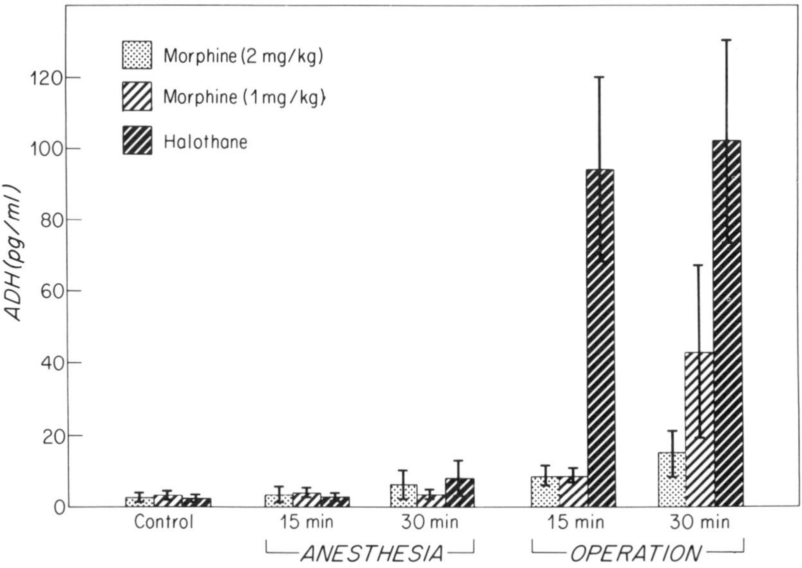

Figure 1. ADH response to anesthesia and surgery. All patients received a 50–50 mixture of oxygen and nitrous oxide. Note that there is no significant increase with anesthesia alone. The response at 30 minutes of surgery was significant for halothane ($p<0.001$) and morphine 1 mg/kg ($p<0.01$), but not for morphine 2 mg/kg.

Other anesthetics such as enflurane [4, 15] and fentanyl[17] have subsequently been studied with similar results. Indeed, the majority of the data support the concept that anesthetics not only do not stimulate the release of ADH but can prevent or obtund such a response to surgical stimulation. It appears that the greater the depth of anesthesia, the less the response to stress stimuli, provided significant hemodynamic changes are not produced. Preliminary data suggest that adequate regional sympathetic blockade can also prevent this ADH response. It is worth noting that in some instances the response to surgery during light anesthesia results in levels of ADH within the range for a significant vasopressor effect. The hypertensive response to skin incision often seen under these conditions may then be due to a vasopressin as well as a cathecholamine response. Recalling the action of ADH on the coronary vascular bed, it is interesting to speculate about the effect of such a high level in patients with clinically significant preexisting coronary artery disease. It is certainly within the realm of possiblity that the evidence of myocardial ischemia and acute left ventricular dysfunction that can appear following such a hypertensive response may be a result of not only increased myocardial oxygen demand but also a decrease in supply availability owing to constriction of the coronary vascular bed.

The levels of ADH required to produce a diuretic-natriuretic response in man are unknown. Recent work from this laboratory suggests that levels beyond the 70 to 100 pg/ml range are required for such an effect.[12] Such concentrations are uncommon and to date have only been demonstrated to occur during cardiopulmonary bypass. Under such a condition, however, a marked increase in urine flow and a substantial Na^+ diuresis were noted, with urinary Na^+ levels rising to 127 mEq/L. Whether such an effect can be demonstrated in other circumstances remains to be determined.

A syndrome of inappropriate secretion of antidiuretic hormone that is usually seen in elderly patients following anesthesia and surgery has also been reported.[1] This appears to be a relatively rare phenomenon and is generally characterized by low serum osmolality, hyponatremia, a variety of neurologic symptoms ranging from restlessness to coma, and the excretion of a hypertonic urine. The precise etiology is unknown, but it is highly unlikely that the anesthetic itself plays any significant role. At any rate, fluid restriction will generally reverse the process in a relatively short period of time.

SUMMARY

Arginine vasopressin, the antidiuretic hormone in man, in low concentrations increases reabsorption of water in the collecting ducts of the kidney, producing a concentrated urine. It is also a potent vasoconstrictor because of its direct effect on arteriolar smooth muscle, particularly the splanchnic, renal, and coronary vascular beds. This appears to be a dose-dependent response. In very high concentrations it is capable of producing a diuresis with increased urinary sodium excretion.

The preponderance of evidence today has failed to show any significant increase in antidiuretic hormone levels with anesthesia alone, provided significant hemodynamic changes do not occur. It seems unlikely, then, that the inhalation anesthetics or high-dose narcotic anesthesia are a direct stimulus to ADH release. If a decrease in urine flow does occur, it is more likely caused by either the renal hemodynamic effects of the anesthetic or a secondary release of ADH. Surgical stimulation is capable of significantly increasing ADH levels. This apparently is a stress response that can be attenuated by the depth of anesthesia. Such a response to operation may produce ADH levels that can indeed decrease urinary flow, but more importantly may succeed in achieving levels that can exert a significant vasopressor effect. In unusual circumstances, vasopressin levels can occur that are capable of producing a diuresis and increased urine sodium excretion.

REFERENCES

1. Deutsch, S., Goldberg, M., and Dripps, R. D.: *Postoperative hyponatremia with the inappropriate release of antidiuretic hormone.* Anesthesiology 27:250–256, 1966.
2. Duke, H. N., Pickford, M., and Watt, J. A.: *The antidiuretic action of morphine: its site and mode of action.* Q. J. Exp. Physiol. 36:149–158, 1951.
3. Glick, S. M., and Haas, M.: *Plasma vasopressin (VP) alterations with surgery.* Proc. Vth Int. Cong. Endocrinol. p. 196, 1976.
4. Hill, G. E., Stanley, T. H., Hodges, M. R., et al.: *Failure of enflurane in altering renal response to acute intracranial pressure increases.* Anesth. Analg. 57:200–205, 1978.
5. Johnson, M. D., Park, C. S., and Malvin, R. L.: *Antidiuretic hormone and the redistribution of renal cortical blood flow.* Am. J. Physiol. 232:F111–F116, 1977.
6. Knight, T., and Weinman, E. J.: *Effect of pharmacologic doses of vasopressin on sodium and water reabsorption in the rat kidney.* Clin. Res. 25:404A, 1976.
7. Kurtzman, N. A., Rogers, P. W., Boonjareen, S., et al.: *Effect of infusion of pharmacologic amounts of vasopressin on renal electrolyte excretion.* Am. J. Physiol. 228:890–894, 1975.
8. Monos, E., Cox, R. H., and Peterson, L. H.: *Direct effects of physiological doses of arginine vasopressin on the arterial wall in vivo.* Am. J. Pysiol. 234:H167–H172, 1978.
9. Moran, W. H., Jr.: *CPPB and vasopressin secretion (editorial).* Anesthesiology 34:501–504, 1971.
10. Morton, J. J., Padfield, P. N., and Forsling, M.: *A radioimmunoassay for plasma arginine vasopressin in man and dog: application to physiological and pathological states.* J. Endocrinol. 65:411–424, 1975.
11. Philbin, D. M., and Coggins, C. H.: *Plasma antidiuretic hormone lev-*

els in cardiac surgical patients during morphine and halothane anesthesia. Anesthesiology 49:95–98, 1978.
12. Philbin, D. M., Coggins, C. H., Emerson, C. W., et al.: *Plasma vasopressin levels and urinary sodium excretion during cardiopulmonary bypass.* J. Thorac. Cardiovasc. Surg. 77:582–589, 1979.
13. Philbin, D. M., Coggins, C. H., Wilson, N., et al.: *Antidiuretic hormone levels during cardiopulmonary bypass.* J. Thorac. Cardiovasc. Surg. 73:145–148, 1977.
14. Philbin, D. M., Wilson, N. E., Sokoloski, J., et al.: *Radioimmunoassay of antidiuretic hormone during morphine anaesthesia.* Can. Anaesth. Soc. J. 23:290–295, 1976.
15. Oyama, T., Taniguchi, K., Ishihara, H., et al.: *Effects of enflurane anesthesia and surgery on endocrine function in man.* Br. J. Anaesth. 51:141–149, 1979.
16. Simpson, P., and Forsling, M.: *The effects of halothane on plasma vasopressin during cardiopulmonary bypass.* Clin. Endocrinol. 7:33–39, 1979.
17. Stanley, T. H., Philbin, D. M., and Coggins, C. H.: *Fentanyl-oxygen anesthesia for coronary artery surgery.* Can. Anaesth. Soc. J. 26:168–172, 1979.
18. Trimble, H. G., and Wood, J. R.: *Pulmonary hemorrhage: its control by the use of intravenous pituitrin.* Dis. Chest 18:345–351, 1950.
19. Wen, S. F. *The effect of vasopressin on phosphate transport in the proximal tubule of the dog.* J. Clin. Invest. 53:660–664, 1974.

5

PREOPERATIVE MANAGEMENT OF THE DIABETIC PATIENT

David G. Johnson, M.D., and
Rubin Bressler, M.D.

A study done several years ago at Temple University indicated that the two principal causes of death in the diabetic patient in the perioperative period are sepsis and complications of arteriosclerosis. Drs. Johnson and Bressler, diabetologists, describe methods for preparing and treating the diabetic patient preoperatively in order to reduce the number and severity of such lethal complications.

Burnell R. Brown, Jr.

Care of the diabetic patient before surgery is important and can be a critical factor in the ultimate outcome of the operative procedure.[3, 4, 7, 8] The two general areas that must be evaluated are the patient's current metabolic status and the chronic effects of diabetes on important organ systems, including the cardiovascular system, the urinary tract, and the nervous system. After evaluation, all measures should be taken to correct reversible abnormalities and compensate for established disability.

Obesity is a frequent accompaniment of adult onset diabetes mellitus that predisposes to many surgical complications. The thick layer of subcutaneous fat can make surgical exposure difficult and increases the problems of wound closure. Loss of mobility caused by obesity may interfere with a patient's ability to change positions in bed, leading to thrombophlebitis of the lower extremities, pulmonary atelectasis, and decubitus ulcers. Therefore, obese diabetic patients in need of elective surgery should be given calorically-restricted diets and the surgery postponed until the patient's regular physician, surgeon, and anesthesiologist are agreed that further delay would be hazardous or unlikely to achieve better control.

Dietary strategies must be adjusted for each patient, based upon his or her motivation, knowledge of nutrition, and cultural and social habits. Nevertheless, the main emphasis in treating obese diabetic patients should be to reduce caloric intake drastically (less than 1200 calories a day) with lesser regard for the long-term nutritional adequacies of the diet or the frequency and pattern of meals. In treating a large number of patients from different backgrounds, we employ various dietary techniques to achieve weight loss, including short periods of total fasting, modified vegans diets, and liquid formula diets. The vegans diet that we prescribe consists of unlimited amounts of raw or cooked vegetables except peas, beans, corn, and potatoes. Limited quantities of fruit, cold cereals (without milk), margarine, peas, beans, seeds, and nuts are also allowed. Bread, meat, milk, milk products, rice, and alcoholic beverages are either excluded or allowed in only very restricted amounts. The liquid formula diets consist of two to three feedings a day of a balanced liquid formula that contains approximately 250 to 300 calories, chiefly in the form of carbohydrate and protein with vitamin supplementation. These more radical methods should be used when patients are unsuccessful in following calorically restricted diets of the American Diabetic Association type.

Most patients with known diabetes should be admitted 1 or 2 days before elective surgery to evaluate their metabolic status and make any necessary adjustments. If routine preoperative tests on a patient disclose the presence of previously undiagnosed diabetes, a similar period of evaluation should occur before any nonemergent operation. Fasting and 2-hour postprandial blood glucose should be measured in addition to serum creatinine and electrolytes. Visual inspection of the plasma will usually reveal significant lipemia, which may signify poor diabetic control or the concurrent existence of pancreatitis. Urine samples should be collected several times daily (such as before meals and at bedtime) to assess glycosuria and the presence of ketones. The overall level of blood glucose control can be estimated by measurement of a 24-hour urine collection for total glucose. The glycosylated hemoglobin concentration (hemoglobin A_{Ic}) provides another index of the degree of previous blood glucose control, since higher concentrations are associated with poorer diabetic control.[1, 2, 5]

Patients in poor diabetic control, as manifested by marked hyperglycemia, dehydration, acidosis, ketonemia, or significant ketonuria should be treated vigorously with insulin, fluids, and strict dietary control to restore optimal metabolic balance before surgery. In general, elective surgery should be postponed until the best possible regulation of the blood sugar, fluid balance, and electrolytes can be achieved.

ASSESSMENT OF CHRONIC COMPLICATIONS OF DIABETES

Diabetes is one of the major diseases that predispose patients to early development of atherosclerosis. Therefore, older patients with diabetes should be questioned about recent chest pain, dyspnea, or palpitations. The general level of physical fitness should be evaluated by questions regarding the regularity and vigor of exercise. If the history or physical examination suggests cardiovascular or respiratory disease, further laboratory tests should be ordered. In addition to the routine EKG and chest x-ray, exercise stress testing, EKG monitoring, or pulmonary function tests may be indicated to rule out or document the severity of myocardial ischemia, myocardial conduction abnormalities, and cardiorespiratory reserve.

In addition to diabetic nephropathy, diabetic patients are at greater risk for the development of other urinary tract problems, including papillary necrosis and atonic bladder. Any abnormalities detected in the initial laboratory tests of serum creatinine or urinalysis should be investigated with further studies, such as urine cultures, creatinine clearance, and 24-hour urinary protein determinations. Radiocontrast studies are hazardous to renal function in diabetics and should be performed only if absolutely necessary. Bladder catheterization can introduce infectious organisms and should be avoided if at all possible.

The neurologic complications of diabetes involve many aspects of neurologic function that can present special problems in the preoperative patient. Autonomic neuropathy may cause vasomotor instability, manifested by orthostatic hypotension. This can be important for surgery performed with the patient in unusual positions. Gastric atony from neuropathy of the visceral nerves may cause nausea, vomiting, and distention, particularly in patients confined in bed. Peripheral and cranial neuropathies interfere with neurologic signs commonly monitored in surgical patients, such as pupillary changes, deep tendon reflexes, and response to pain.

INSULIN THERAPY

Patients with insulin-dependent diabetes mellitus should be given insulin in dosage, form, and time intervals to optimize preoperative glucose control. Usually this is best achieved by giving insulin twice daily in subcutaneous injections that include some intermediate-acting insulin (NPH or lente). If the glucose control is extremely erratic, subcutaneous injections of regular insulin can be given four times daily, based on the patient's anticipated requirements and frequent assessment of the urine and plasma glucose.[10] Typically, one third of the total daily insulin dosage might be given before breakfast, one sixth before lunch, one third before dinner, and one sixth before a small bedtime snack. Urine samples collected during the time periods between insulin injections are tested for total glucose. Insulin dosage can then be adjusted on subsequent days to minimize glucosuria. For example, if the patient spills large amounts of glucose in the urine after lunch, the amount of insulin given just prior to lunch should be increased. A less accurate but more convenient estimate of the pattern of glycosuria can be obtained by measuring the glucose concentration of urine specimens collected just prior to each insulin dose. In this context, it has been common practice previously to administer regular insulin according to a retrospective quantification in which the amount of regular insulin given subcutaneously every 4 to 6 hours is based on the concentration of glucose in the urine tested just prior to each insulin dose. A disadvantage of this technique is that the amount of insulin given is based on the previous blood glucose rather than the anticipated needs for insulin over the subsequent 4 to 6 hours. Obviously this method also requires that the patient have an adequate urine output to permit collection of frequent specimens as well as a normal renal threshold for glucose.

Occasionally patients scheduled for surgery will have extremely variable blood glucose concentrations. Under these circumstances it may be preferable to administer insulin continuously through a subcutaneous or intravenous needle attached to a pump-driven infusion system.[6, 9] The rate of infusion is increased for a short period before meals to compensate for the increased postprandial requirements. Blood glucose is monitored by repetitive blood sampling from an indwelling intravenous pediatric scalp vein or catheter. The glucose concentration can be measured at bedside using a rapid analyzer.

Diabetic patients who do not need insulin ordinarily should have their urine checked frequently for sugar and ketones during the preoperative period to detect the earliest appearance of ketoacidosis, which can intervene during periods of stress. Sulfonylurea agents should be discontinued at least a day before anticipated surgery. This is particularly important in the case of chlorpropamide, which has a duration of action as long as 60 hours. Excretion of chlorpropamide is slowed even further in patients with renal failure. Patients taking sulfonylurea agents who must undergo emergent surgery should be given an intravenous infusion of glucose throughout the period of anesthesia.

The restrictions in diet that are so often necessary before surgery, such as abdominal operations, must be given primary importance. Nevertheless, a well-balanced diabetic diet similar to that which the patient has been following before hospitalization should be prescribed as far as possible. This is particularly true for the insulin-dependent patient, who may require between-meal or bedtime snacks in addition to regular meals.

On the day of surgery, insulin-requiring diabetics should be given less insulin than their usual dose and an intravenous infusion of 5 percent dextrose in water should be given at a rate of approximately 1 liter every $1\frac{1}{2}$ to 2 hours for an adult. For example, if a patient has been receiving a combination of NPH and regular insulin each morning and evening, the morning dose would be reduced to one third or one half the usual dosage. If the patient has been receiving regular insulin every 4 to 6 hours, the insulin dose before surgery should be reduced to 5 to 7 units for an adult.

Whenever possible, surgery on diabetic patients should be performed early in the day, so that the period of lower insulin dosage can be kept as short as possible. This also permits easier monitoring of the patient's status during and after the surgery, with the support of regular laboratory and nursing personnel.

The main goal of preoperative care of the diabetic patient is to prepare him or her for the most successful and least stressful surgery. However, the preoperative period is often a very good time to assess how much patients understand about diabetes and what they should be doing to take care of themselves. As the various tests of organ function, such as stress tests of the heart, are performed, an opportunity is created to discuss with the patient the effects of diabetes on that particular body organ. In hospitals staffed with professional personnel specializing in diabetes, the preoperative period can be used to instruct the patient in various aspects of diabetes care, such as measuring urine glucose and acetone, insulin injection techniques, foot care, and diet. Although the problems of managing the diabetic patient before, during, and after surgery have been treated separately in this book, in actual practice it is essential that there be as smooth and continuous a transition between these various phases as possible. In this era of specialization in medicine it is particularly important that the care of the individual diabetic patient be coordinated closely in all stages by a familiar, preferably small, group of health professionals.

REFERENCES

1. Cerami, A., Koenig, R., and Peterson, C. M.: *Haemoglobin A_{Ic} and diabetes mellitus.* Br. J. Haematol. 38:1, 1978.
2. Gabbay, K. H., Hasty, K., Breslow, J. L., et al.: *Glycosylated hemoglobins and long-term blood glucose control in diabetes mellitus.* J. Clin. Endocrinol. Metab. 44:859, 1977.
3. Galloway, J. A., and Shuman, C. R.: *Profile, specific methods of management, and response of diabetic patients to anesthesia and surgery.* Int. Anesth. Clin. 5:437, 1967.
4. Marble, A., and Steinke, J.: *Guiding the diabetic patient through the surgical period.* Anesthesiology 24:442, 1963.
5. Peterson, C. M., Jones, R. L., Koenig, R. J., et al.: *Reversible hemoglobin sequelae of diabetes mellitus.* Ann. Intern. Med. 86:425, 1977.
6. Santiago, J. V., Clemens, A. H., Clarke, W. L., et al.: *Closed-loop and open-loop devices for blood glucose control in normal and diabetic subjects.* Diabetes 28:71, 1979.
7. Shipp, J.: *Diabetes mellitus, anesthesia, and surgery.* Int. Anesth. Clin. 6:189, 1968.
8. Steinke, J.: *Management of diabetes mellitus and surgery.* N. Engl. J. Med. 282:1472, 1970.
9. Tamborlane, W. V., Sherwin, R. S., Genel, M., et al.: *Administration of insulin to juvenile diabetics via portable pump.* N. Engl. J. Med. 300:573, 1979.
10. Wildberger, H. L., and Ricketts, H. T.: *Multiple injections of crystalline insulin in treatment of labile diabetes.* J.A.M.A. 172:655, 1960.

6

CENTRAL DIABETES INSIPIDUS

John H. Finley, M.D.

Dr. Finley discusses some of the vicissitudes of the anesthetic management of patients with diabetes insipidus. There is no specific anesthetic or technique that can be considered better than any other in this endocrinopathy. Rather, a basic knowledge of pathophysiology of the disease is the paramount consideration.

Burnell R. Brown, Jr.

Diabetes insipidus is a syndrome characterized by the inability to conserve water either by a central mechanism (a deficiency in vasopressin release) or a nephrogenic mechanism (lack of response to vasopressin in the tubules). This discussion will mainly be limited to central diabetes insipidus (CDI).

ETIOLOGY

The causes of CDI are varied. The most common lesions are intracerebral tumors.[5] These tumors may originate in the brain as pituitary adenoma, craniopharyngioma, pinealoma, and glioma; or may be metastatic or infiltrative (leukemia). If the lesion itself does not cause CDI, the removal of the tumor many times will. This occurs when more than 85 percent of the supraoptic or paraventricular cell bodies or neurons are destroyed.[1]

There are other conditions associated with CDI. These are intracerebral hemorrhage, severe head trauma to the basilar areas of the skull, Hand-Schuller-Christian disease, infectious disease, congenital malformations, vascular disorders, and some of the granulomatous diseases.[2] Hypophysectomy for metastatic breast carcinoma may also be associated with CDI. There is also a small group of patients with what in the past has been called idiopathic CDI. It has been shown on postmortem examination that most, but not all, have some kind of pituitary or hypothalamic lesion.

PATHOPHYSIOLOGY

Antidiuretic hormone (ADH) is an octapeptide formed in the supraoptic nuclei of the hypothalamus. It is carried by a large protein molecule (neurophysin) down the neurons of the pituitary. ADH is disengaged from neurophysin in the posterior lobe and released into the circulation by various stimuli. Stimuli include changes in blood volume or osmolality, pain, emotional stress, certain drugs, and activation of aortic baroreceptors.

Once ADH is in the circulation, it is bound to the contraluminal side of the collecting duct of the nephron. It interacts with adenyl cyclase to form cyclic AMP, which in turn stimulates protein kinase on the intraluminal side. Protein kinase induces phosphorylation of membrane proteins. This causes an increase in permeability of the membrane with increased absorption of free water from the duct. The process can be inhibited by hypokalemia, hypercalcemia, and prostaglandin E.[3]

During normal daily function, osmotic changes are the major mechanism for release of ADH. Osmolality is normally maintained in a very narrow range (2 percent change between diuresis and antidiuresis).[3] In CDI, ADH is missing and there is a corresponding lack of osmolar control. This can lead to tremendous losses of free water with hypernatremia and dehydration. The volume response with ADH can work synergistically or antagonistically with osmotic response. In dehydration with water loading, both factors work together, while in hypotonic hypovolemia, the osmotic effect is overidden by volume effect.

Lesions causing the CDI syndrome can occur at three levels:

1. There may be a defect in the osmoreceptors of the hypothalamus. The receptors can be set too high, i.e., above 287 mOsm/L, or may be completely nonfunctioning. In many cases the ADH response to other mechanisms causing release will still be intact.

2. The lesion may be one that occurs in the supraoptic nuclei or supraoptic-neurohypophyseal tract. Interruption of the neurohypophyseal tract must occur above the median eminence for it to be of consequence. Otherwise, ADH will continue to be released at the end of the transected neurons. The different tumors causing CDI most commonly have their effect at this level. Also, severe basilar skull trauma probably causes disruption of nerve axons. This may or may not be reversible.

3. The effect may occur at the storage site of vasopressin. This may also be part of the mechanism for inherited CDI, a Mendelian dominant disease.

CLINICAL FINDINGS

The main clinical findings in diabetes insipidus are polyuria and polydipsia. The urine is dilute and pale and may reach 20 liters per day in extreme cases. Patients will show signs of dehydration: poor skin turgor, dry skin, constipation, and intense thirst. Even with severe water deprivation these patients still have polyuria that will continue until vascular collapse.

Acute CDI after surgery, trauma, or cerebral vascular accidents may show several patterns.[5] Cerebral edema in the postinjury period starts at 12 to 24 hours and is maximal at 48 to 72 hours. The degree of damage caused by the edema is variable. The lesion must be high on the pituitary stalk or at the supraoptic nuclei for the patient to show symptoms of CDI. Clinically, different degrees of polyuria may be seen, depending on the amount of damage done. Prognosis is variable and cannot usually be estimated from the degree of polyuria alone.

There are four distinct syndromes seen in the postoperative or traumatic patient:

1. The most common starts within 24 to 72 hours and may last a week. This type is transient and patients will undergo a full recovery. It is probably secondary to edema at the level of the hypothalamus.

2. In the triphasic syndrome the patient is polyuric, initially secondary to edema, but within a few days returns to normal. This in turn is followed by permanent CDI. The lesion involved is transection of pituitary stalk with some residual ADH available.

3. The third syndrome is polyuria, which begins at 24 to 72 hours after surgery but then decreases as brain edema is reduced. The patient never completely returns to normal ADH output.

4. The fourth syndrome starts 24 to 72 hours after surgery and is permanent without any improvement.

DIAGNOSIS

Differential diagnosis of CDI includes consideration of psychogenic polydipsia, chronic nephritis, diabetes mellitus, hypochloremic alkalosis, hypercalcemia, vitamin D intoxication, and nephrogenic diabetes insipidus (NDI).[1] A simple determination of a blood glucose, calcium, potassium, and pH can eliminate most of these. Nephritis can be ruled out by the lack of protein and cells in the urine. The difficult differential diagnosis is between NDI, psychogenic polydipsia, and CDI. Discriminatory examinations include:

Dehydration Test

Patients are kept without water for 6 to 18 hours. In normal patients the urine volume decreases to 1 ml/min with decreased excretion of free water. This occurs over 4 to 6 hours. Patients with diabetes insipidus will continue to excrete hypoosmolar urine. They may lose up to 3 kg of body weight. Patients with partial CDI will show some concentrating ability but will still have free water excretion.[3]

Vasopressin Test

This is employed after the dehydration test, if the patient is still polyuric. It consists of administration of vasopressin 5 units I.C. and observance of whether there are changes in the urinary osmolality. In CDI there will be an increase in the concentration of urine within 1 to 2 hours. Patients with intrinsic kidney disease will have no change in urine osmolality.[1]

Hypertonic Saline Test

This test depends upon infusions of 2.5 or 5 percent saline. It is cumbersome and less reliable than the water deprivation test.[3]

Measurements of Urinary and Blood ADH

These tests are usually not needed except for a very difficult diagnostic case.

Nicotine Test

This rarely used test consists of giving patients nicotine (through smoking), which in turn stimulates the supraoptic nuclei, causing antidiuresis. This does not occur in CDI.[1]

After trauma or surgery the diagnosis may be more difficult and critical than with patients with chronic CDI. These patients often have received large amounts of fluids during the operation or after injury. This may lead to a confusing clinical picture, especially if they are incontinent and do not have a urinary catheter. Diagnosis is made by a high degree of clinical suspicion and careful observation of fluid and electrolyte balance.

TREATMENT

The most common drugs used in treatment of CDI are the various vasopressin derivatives. Aqueous vasopressin has a relatively short duration of action (4–6 hours). It can either be used in a single injection or continuous intravenous infusion. Pitressin (tannate-in-oil) has a longer duration, approximately 24 to 72 hours. It is most often used in long-term outpatient therapy. There are two synthetic derivatives that can be used as a nasal spray. Lysine vasopressin is the shorter acting of the two, with a duration of 6 to 8 hours. The newer agent 1-desamino-8-arginine vasopressin is longer acting (12 hours).[4] ADH derivatives must be used carefully. Some patients who are sensitive to the drug may show extreme degrees of fluid retention with normal doses. Therefore, a small test dose is usually given. A relative contraindication to the exogenous hormone is coronary artery and peripheral vascular disease, since the drug has been associated with vascular spasm. Allergic reactions with the drugs are common. Patients may be desensitized if the allergy is serious.

Nonpituitary preparations are occasionally used in the chronic treatment of mild CDI when only a small concentration of endogenous ADH is present. Chlorpropamide, the oral hypoglycemic, will often decrease polyuria. The disulfiram-like symptoms and hypoglycemia may cause difficulty with patient acceptance. Other compounds used to treat CDI are carbamazepine, vincristine, cyclophosphamide, clofibrate, and acetaminophen. All of these increase endogenous ADH release.[3]

In the patient with chronic CDI who can take fluids orally, treatment is not an emergency. Given one or a combination of the above drugs, almost all patients with CDI can be well controlled. Therapy should be instituted carefully.

ANESTHESIA CONSIDERATIONS

Preoperatively the patient's fluid status should be evaluated carefully. If needed, he should be appropriately hydrated before elective surgery. Baseline weight electrolytes, hematocrit, BUN, and plasma osmolality should be obtained in patients with CDI or at a high risk for developing it. If the patients have CDI preoperatively, antidiuretic therapy should be continued to the time of surgery. During surgery a patient with CDI is usually not a severe clinical problem if vasopressin is given preoperatively. If polyuria does occur, replacement should be with free water plus appropriate treatment of surgical losses. Aqueous vasopressin can be used. Some patients will retain water secondary to preoperative medication. In these patients normal saline must be used to counteract the hyponatremia. In all cases electrolytes should be drawn at intervals during surgery, and urinary output needs to be monitored with an indwelling catheter. Postoperative management of the patient should be planned according to the clinical course. In patients with preoperative CDI, improvement after surgery is rare. They should resume preoperative medications as soon as practical.

The patients who are at high risk for developing CDI postoperatively should be monitored closely. Urine output is followed with an indwelling catheter or close nursing supervision. Urine specific gravity should be measured every 3 to 4 hours. Serum electrolytes, BUN, and osmolarity are drawn every other day until polyuria starts. The patient's weight is obtained at least daily.

If polyuria appears, treatment depends on the patient's status. If he is alert and able to take fluids by mouth, the patient can usually regulate his own fluid management. Careful input and output records must be kept. The need for laboratory work (e.g., electrolytes) will increase initially to at least twice a day until the patient stabilizes. If he cannot maintain adequate intake, aqueous vasopressin can be started. When the patient has stabilized he may be changed to long-term therapy, if needed.

In the patients who are obtunded or lethargic, the diagnosis of CDI may be more difficult. Usually, continued diuresis in the face of a rising hematocrit, sodium, and osmolality with a dilute urine will differentiate these patients from those with simple postoperative diuresis. Once the diagnosis is made, CDI patients are treated again with intravenous fluids and vasopressin. Fluids are dextrose in water solutions with a liter of balanced electrolyte daily. Replacement is calculated by insensible plus urinary loss. It is important to watch for water intoxication manifested by lethargy, confusion, seizures, and coma.

It must be remembered that many if not most patients with acute CDI will improve. Therapy in these patients should be predicated on this assumption.

REFERENCES

1. Dingman, J., and Thorn, G.: "Diseases of the neurohypophysis." In Wintrobe, M. M., et al. (eds.): *Harrison's Principles of Internal Medicine.* ed. 7. McGraw-Hill, New York, 1974.
2. Michael, U. F.: Polyuric Syndromes. Ariz. Med. 4:269–273, April 1978.
3. Moses, A. M., Myron, M., and Streetin, D. H. P.: *Pathophysiologic and pharmacologic alterations in the release and action of ADH.* Metabolism 25:697–721, 1976.
4. Robinson, A. G.: *ADAVP in the treatment of central diabetes insipidus.* N. Engl. J. Med. 294:507–511, 1976.
5. Shucart, W. A., and Jackson, I.: *Management of diabetes insipidus in the neurosurgical patients.* Neurosurg. 44:65–71, 1976.

7

EFFECTS OF ANESTHESIA AND SURGERY ON THYROID FUNCTION

Simon Halevy, M.D.

In this detailed chapter, Dr. Halevy minutely describes the effects of anesthetics on thyroid function. He synthesizes the newest information available concerning this important endocrine organ. Comprehension of these physiologic events will yield the anesthesiologist a great deal of insight into assessing patients with thyroid dysfunction for anesthesia.

Burnell R. Brown, Jr.

The main function of the thyroid gland is to secrete thyroid hormones, which are extremely important in growth and development and the maturation of the central nervous system in the perinatal period. They are important in carbohydrate metabolism and synthesis and metabolism of proteins and lipids. Thyroid hormones also play a major role in oxygen consumption and thermogenesis. In addition, the thyroid hormones have the capacity to influence other hormones, drug metabolism, and various metabolic pathways.[54] The thyroid hormones are iodinated thyroglobulins. The synthesis of primary thyroglobulins, monoiodotyrosine (MIT) and diiodotyrosine (DIT), takes place in the thyroid gland from amino acids, hexoses, and oxidized iodine (Fig. 1).[18, 30, 53, 72]

Plasma supplies iodide, which is mainly of dietary origin. Iodide becomes thyroid iodide by the process of uptake or trap-

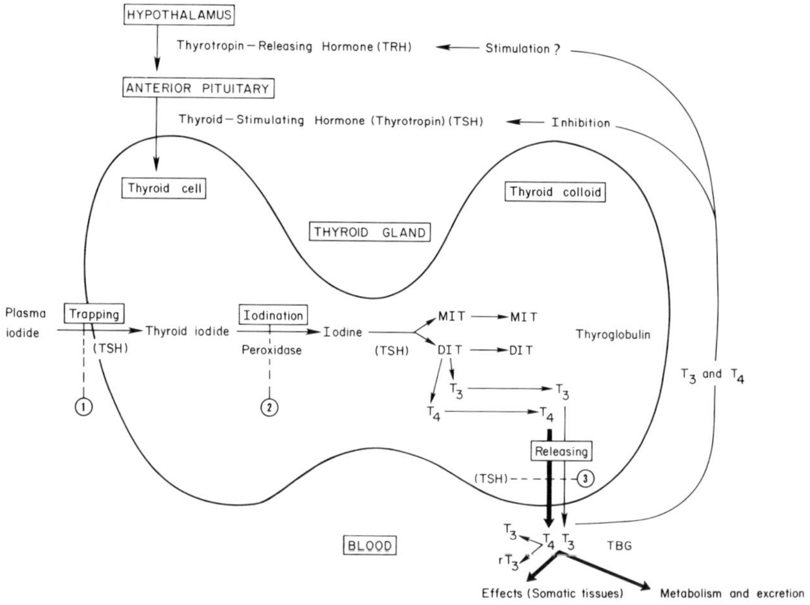

Figure 1. Summary of thyroid hormones pathway. TSH = thyrotropin-dependent process. 1–3 = main inhibition sites; inhibited by (1) perchlorate, thiocyanate, methimazole; (2) thiouracil; (3) iodide, lithium. MIT = 3-monoidotyrosine. DIT = 3,5-diiodotyrosine. TBG = thyronine-binding globulin. T_4 = 3,5,3′,5′-tetraiodothyronine (thyroxine). T_3 = 3,5,3′-triiodothyronine, rT_3 = 3,3′,5′-triiodothyronine (reverse T_3).

ping, which depends on the thyroid-stimulating hormone (thyrotropin, TSH), and is further oxidized to iodine during the process of iodination with the help of an enzyme (peroxidase). The main thyroid hormones, 3,5,3′,5′-tetraiodothyronine (thyroxine, T_4) and 3,5,3′-triiodothyronine (T_3), originate from the primary thyroglobulins, MIT and DIT, by the process of coupling. An essential amino acid, tyrosine, combines with iodine to form mostly T_4, but also T_3, which are then stored as thyroglobulins. All thyroglobulins are contained in the intrafollicular colloid of the thyroid gland. Particles of this colloid are ingested by the thyroid cells. Subsequently, free (unbound to protein) T_4 and T_3 are secreted and released into the circulation, where they are mostly bound to a plasma protein, thyronine-binding globulin (TBG), and represent the active circulating form of thyroid hormones. Both are metabolized by the liver and the kidney and ultimately either excreted or changed into free, that is, unbound hormones. Unbound hormones are the only forms that enter various tissues and exert the physiologic activity of thyroid hormones. The most important active thyroid hormone is T_3.[45, 74] This hormone, together with another, recently discovered thyroid hormone, 3,3′,5′-triiodothyronine (reverse T_3 or rT_3), considered to be inactive, is mostly produced in the periphery, that is, outside the thyroid gland, by the monodeiodination of T_4.

The hypothalamus secretes a neurohormone, thyrotropin-releasing hormone (TRH), which stimulates the secretion of the pituitary TSH (thyroid-stimulating hormone). TSH performs multiple functions, such as stimulation of iodide uptake by the thyroid gland, stimulation of the synthesis of thyroid hormones, the breakdown of thyroglobulins in the thyroid cell, and finally the secretion of free T_4 and T_3 (Fig. 1). In the thyroid cell, TSH stimulates the production of cyclic 3′,5′ adenosine monophosphate (cAMP), which is considered the main mechanism of action of TSH. From this diagrammatic presentation (Fig. 1), it is easy to understand that, at least theoretically, pharmacologic agents, anesthesia, trauma, and surgery may interfere with thyroid processes at any level and therefore alter thyroid function or the blood level of the active thyroid hormones.

The effect of stress on thyroid function has long been recognized. Mice exposed to starvation, cold, heat, and tourniquet stress were found to have low protein-bound iodine in the serum, that is, low thyroxine.[79] Furthermore, a number of environmental factors that exist in the operating room or laboratory, such as temperature, humidity, transfer, noise, light, handling, and injection, play an important role in thyroid activity through a central mechanism.[19, 20, 46] For instance, hypothermia is known to induce TSH release, especially in children and rodents, through TRH secretion.[34, 46, 78] This cold stimulation of TRH, the hypothalamic hormone, in the rat may be blocked by phenobarbital, diethyl ether, and other agents, such as phentolamine, reserpine, and atropine.[43] In addition, other experiments in rats have shown that most anesthetics would reverse the TSH response to cold.[48]

The anesthesiologist needs to know: (1) whether anesthetics, anesthetic techniques, or surgery affects thyroid function or thyroid hormones, (2) if anesthesia has any adverse effects, (3) the intensity and duration of these putative effects, and (4) what is the practical importance of the known scientific data on potential clinical effects of anesthesia on normal or altered thyroid function during pregnancy, early infancy, or the postoperative period.

At the present time, there is no definitive answer to any of these questions for several reasons. Until recently, there has been a lack of sensitive and precise methods for the determination of thyroid hormones and insufficient data concerning the effect of surgery alone on thyroid function, that is, independent of the added effect of anesthesia. There has also been a lack of quantitative studies showing the influence of anesthesia on thyroid hormones in hypothyroidism, in hyperthyroidism, or during other conditions such as pregnancy or the neonatal period, which are associated with physiologic alterations of thyroid function. An important volume of information on thyroid function and hormones is accumulating, and new and interesting data suggest anesthetic effects on thyroid function. However, the significance of the new data to anesthesia practice is difficult to establish at the present time.

In view of these problems, a critical review of clinical and experimental information concerning the effects of anesthesia and surgery on thyroid function and hormones appears necessary and timely. The available bibliographic material on anesthesia and surgery can be organized as follows: (1) effects on thyroid-stimulating hormone, (2) effects on serum thyroxine, (3) effects on triiodothyronine and reverse triiodothyronine production and metabolism, and (4) influence of thyroid hormones on anesthesia or anesthetic action.

EFFECTS OF ANESTHESIA AND SURGERY ON THYROID-STIMULATING HORMONE

Two important aspects will be discussed: iodine uptake and release as a test of thyroid function and TSH activity, and the influence of anesthesia and surgery on serum TSH level.

IODINE UPTAKE AND RELEASE

One of the first laboratory techniques to investigate thyroid function was based on the uptake by an intact thyroid gland or the release by an artificially blocked thyroid of an injected dose of radioactive iodine. Since both these processes are generally under TSH control, this was an indirect test to evaluate hormonal function and thyroid gland response.

A number of animal experiments suggested that barbiturates, especially thiobarbiturates such as thiopental, may acutely depress the uptake of injected radioactive iodine (^{131}I).[42, 52, 71, 76, 77] Wase and Foster showed a dose-related decrease of ^{131}I uptake in the rat following thiopental administration (Table 1).[75] This study demonstrated a quantitative relationship between the effects of anesthesia and thyroid function, although the conclusion suggested lack of a pitutary role in this process. Oyama reported similar findings using cyclopropane, diethyl ether, and thiopental anesthesia.[55, 56] The effect of thiopental was related

Table 1. Four-Hour Uptake of I^{131} by Rat Thyroid in Relation to Amount of Thiopental Administered (2 μC I^{131} intraperitoneally).

Dose (mg/kg)	*I^{131} CPM/mg*	*Percentage*
0	214 ± 19*	100
5	138 ± 15	64.4
10	112 ± 14	52.3
20	76 ± 9	35.5
40	44 ± 7	20.6
70	26 ± 5	12.2

*Standard error of the mean. (From Wase, A. W., and Foster, W. C.: *Thiopental and thyroid metabolism.* Proc. Soc. Exp. Biol. Med. 91:89–91, 1956, with permission.)

to the presence of thiourea structure (HN–C=S–NH) in the thiopental molecule, which is similar to thiouracil, a potent inhibitor of iodination and thyroid hormone synthesis.[1, 49] Oyama was also one of the first to stress the importance of complex endocrine relationships with respect to anesthesia and surgery.[62] However, these studies showed only indirect evidence that TSH may be altered by anesthesia.

In human studies, following surgery and general anesthesia, when thyroid uptake or the release of ^{131}I was measured, both an increase and a decrease were reported.[17, 22, 26, 27, 37] These studies attributed the observed changes mostly to surgery and its complex endocrine and metabolic effects. The decrease in iodine uptake was also attributed to the increase of glucocorticosteroids, which occurred after surgery and diethyl ether or cyclopropane anesthesia.[5, 8, 27, 67] It is possible that altered peripheral distribution of thyroid hormones during anesthesia and surgery could be responsible for these findings, as was suggested by some of the early studies investigating TSH activity.[24]

INFLUENCE OF ANESTHESIA AND SURGERY ON TSH LEVEL

A significant improvement in the study of TSH metabolism was the introduction of direct methods for the measurement of this hormone in the blood. The radioimmunoassay technique (RIA), one of the latest, more sensitive, and reliable methods, has gained widespread acceptance in laboratory determination of the hormone.

When the pituitary thyrotropic hormone was measured (Table 2) in animal experiments following general anesthesia, an increase after pentobarbital and chloral hydrate and a biphasic response after thiopental, diethyl ether, halothane, and methoxyflurane were reported.[48] However, in human studies (with two exceptions) using thiopental, diethyl ether, halothane, or methoxyflurane, no significant changes in TSH levels were detected.[10, 31, 41, 60, 61] Only one study showing similar results used regional (epidural) anesthesia.[31] A biphasic response was reported after neuroleptanalgesia technique for cardiopulmonary bypass[47] and in one study after halothane anesthesia (Table 2).[40]

However, we may conclude from recent studies that general or regional anesthesia does not influence thyrotropin secretion and blood levels in man.[4, 7, 25, 28, 29, 32, 33, 35, 40, 44, 51, 57-59, 63-66, 68, 73]

EFFECTS OF ANESTHESIA AND SURGERY ON SERUM THYROXINE CONCENTRATION

The study of the effects of anesthesia and surgery on thyroxine (T_4) production, metabolism, and blood levels occupies most of the literature in this area.

The perioperative changes in T_4, as well as T_3 and reverse T_3, cannot be accurately evaluated without the concomitant study of protein binding and shift, that is, thyroxine-binding globulin (TBG) changes. Recent studies have shown that the serum levels of these hormones and of TBG may vary because of their continuous exchange between the vascular and extravascular compartments, such as the liver. It is, therefore, necessary to examine two important aspects of thyroxine metabolism: the variations of TBG and other hormone-binding proteins in the serum, and T_4 blood concentration changes under the same conditions.

VARIATIONS OF TBG AND OTHER HORMONE-BINDING PROTEINS IN SERUM

The availability of free hormone, capable of hormonal action at tissue level, depends on the amount of unbound hormone, that is, protein-free hormone. A general formula showing these relationships is applicable to both T_4 and T_3:

$$[FT_4] = \frac{[TBG - T_4]}{[TBG]} = [TBG - T_4] \times [TBG]^{-1}$$

where $[FT_4]$ (or, in the case of T_3, $[FT_3]$) is the serum concentration of free thyroxine (or T_3), and $[TBG - T_4]$ is the serum concentration of the total hormone, bound and unbound. This formula is important since it shows how these factors are interconnected and may influence each other during surgery and other conditions. Similarly, it is well known from general pharmacology that the availability of free drug capable of pharmacologic action depends, among other factors, on the amount of unbound fraction of the drug, that is, the protein-free fraction.

As an application of these principles to the laboratory determination of hormone, one can indirectly measure the amount of hormone by determining the amount of protein binding. A

Table 2. Influence of Anesthesia and Surgery on Serum Thyroid Hormones.

Thyroid Hormone	*Species*	*Primary Anesthetic(s)*	*Technique*
Thyroid stimulating hormone (TSH)	Man	Thiopental-N_2O	
		" Meperidine-diazepam	
		N_2O-fentanyl-phenoperidine	
		Diethyl ether	
		Halothane	
		Methoxyflurane	
		Lidocaine; 2-Chloroprocaine; bupivacaine	Epidural
	Rat	Pentobarbital	i.p.
		Chloral hydrate	
		Urethane	s.c.; i.p.
		Thiopental	i.p.
		Diethyl ether	
		Halothane	
		Methoxyflurane	
Thyroxine (T_4)	Man	?	?
		?	General; subarachnoid block; local
		?	
		?	
		Thiopental	

+ = increased serum concentration
− = decreased serum concentration
0 = no change
NS = not significant
i.p. = intraperitoneal
s.c. = subcutaneous

Response	Maximum Change Δ %	Remarks	References
0		Slight increase (NS)	Oyama[61]
0		Cesarean section	Halevy[31]
Biphasic	+31−15	Cardiopulmonary bypass	McDonald[47]
0		Slight immediate decrease	Oyama[61]
0		Slight immediate decrease	Oyama[60]
+	38	NS	Kirby[41]
Biphasic	+22−78		Kehlet[40]
0		Slight decrease	Oyama[60]
−	19	NS	Halevy[31]
0			Ducommun[19]
+	79		Männistö[48]
+	38		
+	12		
Biphasic	+57−28		
	+11−52		
	+74−31		
	+50−22		
0		SPI method	Engstrom[22]
+	1000	PBI method	Goldenberg[26]
+		PBI method	Goldenberg[28]
−	10		Burr[7]
0		BEI method	Goldenberg[27]
0			Oyama[63]
−	8	PBI method	

SPI = serum-precipitable iodine
PBI = protein-bound iodine
BEI = butanol-extractable iodine
RT_3U = resin triiodothyronine uptake
(SPI, PBI, BEI and RT_3U are methods for indirect thyroxine estimation)
(1) = reversed by thiocyanate (SCN^-)
(2) = A thiobarbiturate

Table 2. Continued

Thyroid Hormone	Species	Primary Anesthetic(s)	Technique
		" N_2O	
		Nitrous oxide	
		Fentanyl-phenoperidine	
		Thiopental-meperidine-diazepam	
		Althesin	
		Diethyl ether	
		Halothane	

Response	Maximum Change Δ %	Remarks	References
0			Oyama[66]
−	12.3		Oyama[65]
0		Slight early decrease (NS)	Oyama[61]
+	125	Free T_4 measured	Surks[73]
+	104	T_4 dialyzable fraction measured	
+	77	Cardiopulmonary bypass	Macdonald[47]
+	23	" "	
		RT_3U method	
−	14	Cesarean section	Halevy[31]
−	5	Total T_4	Oyama[58]
+	9	Free thyroxine index	
0		Thyroid surgery; also local anesthesia	Hydovitz[35]
+	20	NS; also subarachnoid block	Greene[29]
+			Goldenberg[25]
+	180		Fore[24]
+	70	PBI	
+	12.5	RT_3U	
+	40		Oyama[63]
+	14	RT_3U	
+	40		Oyama[66]
+	36		Oyama[61]
+	35.5		Oyama[65]
+		RT_3U	Johnson[37]
+	22	PBI	Oyama[67]
+	27	RT_3U	
+	21.2		Oyama[65]
+	28		Oyama[60]
+	21		Harland[33]
0		PBI	
+	60	Free thyroxine	Kirby[41]
+	23	NS	

Table 2. Continued

Thyroid Hormone	Species	Primary Anesthetic(s)	Technique
		Methoxyflurane	
		Enflurane	
		Isoflurane	
		Tetracaine	Subarachnoid block
		Quatacaine	
		Lidocaine	
		Bupivacaine	Epidural
		Lidocaine; 2-chloroprocaine; bupivacaine	
	Rat	Urethane	i.p.
		Pentobarbital; barbital	
		Pentobarbital	i.p.
		Allobarbital	
		Inactin[2]	
		Innovar Vet.	
		Diethyl ether (light)	Inhalation
		(deep)	i.p.

Response	Maximum Change Δ %	Remarks	References
+	20		Harland[32]
Biphasic	−8+20	Total thyroxine	Kehlet[40]
+	45	Free thyroxine	
0			Oyama[64]
0		RT_3U	
0			Oyama[60]
+	30		Brandt[4]
+	25	RT_3U	
Biphasic	+13−30		Oyama[68]
+	37	Total T_4	Oyama[57]
+	20	RT_3U	
+	69	Free thyroxine index	
+	20		Greene[29]
0			Fore[24]
+	10		Oyama[59]
−	10		
−	20		Brandt[4]
+	20	RT_3U	
−	19	Cesarean section	Halevy[31]
−(1)			Langer[44]
−	33	PBI	Premachandra[71]
−(1)			Langer[44]
−(1)			
+	9	Free T_4	Michajlovskij[51]
+	22	Total T_4	
+	88	Free T_4	
+	29	Total T_4	
−(1)			Langer[44]
−(1)			
−(1)			
−	14	Free T_4	Michajlovskij[51]
+	8	Total T_4	
+	10	Free T_4	
+	31	Total T_4	

Table 2. Continued

Thyroid Hormone	Species	Primary Anesthetic(s)	Technique
Triiodothyronine (T_3)	Man	?	
		N_2O-fentanyl-phenoperidine	
		Thiopental-meperidine-diazepam	
		Halothane	
		Enflurane	
		Bupivacaine	
		Lidocaine; 2-chloroprocaine; bupivacaine	
Reverse triiodothyronine (rT_3)	Man	?	
		Thiopental-meperidine-diazepam	
		Lidocaine; 2-Chloroprocaine bupivacaine	

method known as the resin T_3 uptake determines the available binding sites on the protein TBG. The availability of these binding sites depends on the amount of T_4 or T_3 bound to the protein: a large amount of hormone will evidently occupy more binding sites on the protein molecule. For these reasons, it is expected that if the amount of TBG is increased during pregnancy, or decreased by shifting to other compartments during surgery, the availability of the protein and its binding sites will change. Therefore, the results of hormone determination may not accu-

Response	Maximum Change Δ %	Remarks	References
−	43		Burr[7]
−	55		Macdonald[47]
−	35	Cesarean section	Halevy[31]
+	19	Free T_3	Kirby[41]
−	47	Free T_3	Kehlet[40]
−	50	Total T_3	
−	41		Brandt[4]
Biphasic	+13−30		Oyama[68]
−	33		Brandt[4]
−	32	Cesarean section	Halevy[31]
+	70		Burr[7]
+	11	Cesarean section	Halevy[41]
−	16	" "	

rately reflect the actual change in hormone blood concentration.

In addition, certain drugs, such as thiobarbiturates (thiopental, Inactin), diphenylhydantoin, diazepam, heparin, salicylates, and phenols, may affect hormone binding to protein because they exert competitive binding and sometimes displace the free hormone from its protein-bound association, as they do with other compounds.[44, 51] These mechanisms may interfere with laboratory determination and interpretation of the results, during anesthesia and surgery, and other physiologic and pathologic conditions. Furthermore, other factors such as posture and venous compression with resulting hemoconcentration, in association with surgery, show increased values for both T_3 and T_4 because of the increase in hormone-binding protein (Fig. 2).[38]

Although TBG is the most important serum protein to bind primarily T_4, there are other hormone-binding proteins in the blood. One of the best proteins studied in relation to surgery is the thyroxine-binding prealbumin (TBPA). Surks and Oppenheimer studied surgical patients and showed a decrease in TBPA and an increase in free thyroxine blood level by a mechanism similar to that described in connection with TBG (Fig. 3).[73] No data concerning anesthesia utilized in those cases were presented. However, this study is important since it stresses the importance of serum protein variations in relation to surgery and thyroid hormones. Similar results were recently reported by Bernstein and associates[3] and Kirby and coworkers.[41] One of the major causes of these protein changes in surgical patients is the

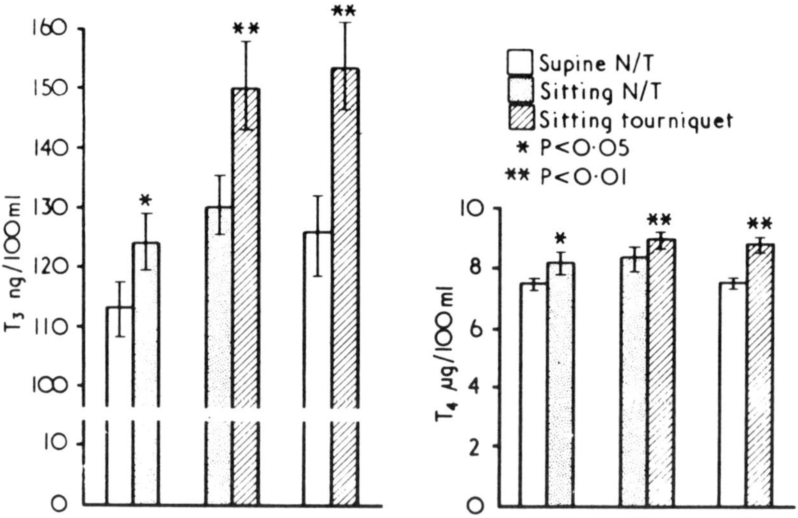

Figure 2. Effect of hemoconcentration of serum levels of triiodothyronine and thyroxine. (From Judd, S. J., Carter, J. N., and Corcoran, J. M.: *Circulating thyroid hormone concentrations and posture and venous compression.* Br. Med. J. 27 Dec.: 735–736, 1975, with permission.)

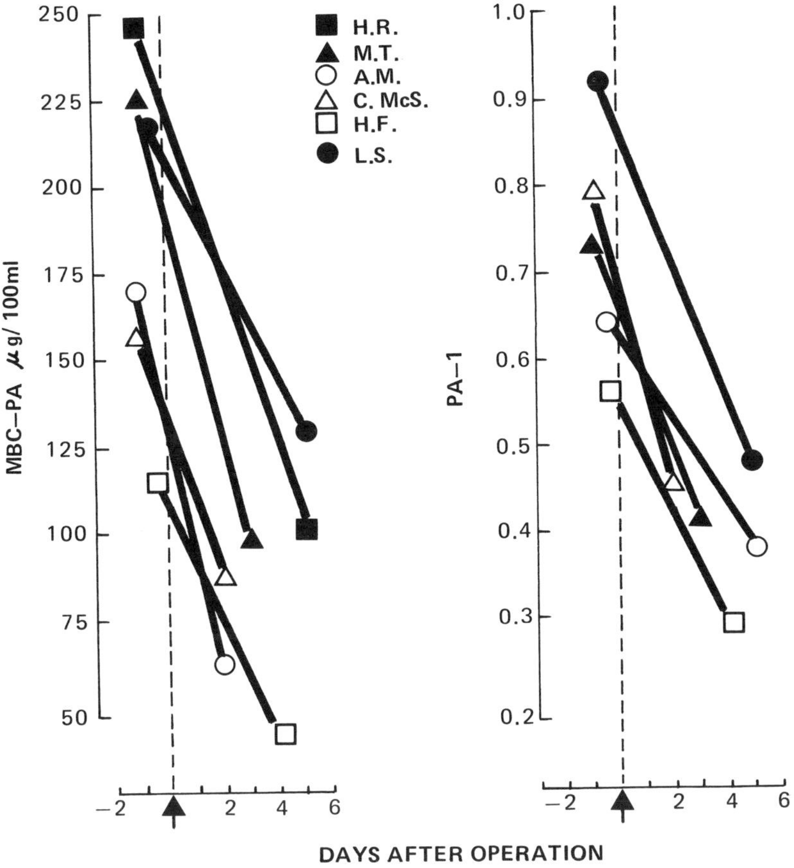

Figure 3. Maximal depression in binding capacity TBPA (MBC-PA) and concentration of PA-1. (From Surks, M. I., and Oppenheimer, J. H.: *Postoperative changes in the concentration of thyroxine-binding prealbumin and serum free thyroxine.* J. Clin. Endocrinol. 24:794–802, 1964, with permission.)

shift of fluids, proteins, and electrolytes between the vascular and extravascular spaces, mainly in the liver.

The variation in T_4 during anesthesia and surgery has also been attributed to the shift of this hormone in and out of the vascular compartment, either alone or bound to serum proteins.[24, 32, 44, 51, 63, 65, 67] The liver is considered the major extravascular organ contributing to this exchange.

BLOOD OR SERUM THYROXINE AND ANESTHESIA

The data presented in Table 2 leads to the following conclusions: With few exceptions, most anesthetics increase T_4 serum level, and some anesthetics, e.g., thiopental and methoxyflurane, consistently decrease or do not change T_4 blood concentrations. Other anesthetics, such as diethyl ether, halothane, and enflurane, are practically always associated with an increase in T_4 blood levels (Table 3, Fig. 4, and Fig. 5).[4, 40] Therefore, it seems that, at least theoretically, anesthetics associated with an increase in T_4 blood levels should not be used in cases of hyperthyroidism. Data concerning other general anesthetics are insufficient.

Regional anesthesia and local anesthetics probably do not change or minimally decrease T_4 in the blood (Fig. 4 and Fig. 6).[4, 31]

Some of the data are contradictory in part because different laboratory methods were used for T_4 estimation: indirect methods such as SPI, PBI, BEI, and RT_3U (Table 2), and direct methods such as radioimmunoassay.

The few animal studies use only the rat. One study demonstrates differential effects between light and deep diethyl ether anesthesia and a significant increase of T_4 after inactin anesthesia, which is a thiobarbiturate (Fig. 7).[51]

A number of studies do not mention the anesthetic used, assuming that surgery alone influences T_4 blood or serum levels (Fig. 8).[7] Surgery may be associated with a shift of T_4 from nonvascular spaces.[24] This may cause the increase of T_4 in blood levels after most anesthetics.

EFFECTS OF ANESTHESIA AND SURGERY ON TRIIODOTHYRONINE AND REVERSE TRIIODOTHYRONINE PRODUCTION, BLOOD LEVEL AND METABOLISM

The influence of anesthesia and surgery on the production of T_3 and rT_3 is of scientific and practical interest. These hormones are metabolic products resulting from the peripheral, that is, outside the thyroid gland, monodeiodination of thyroxine, mostly in the liver and kidney. Only a small part of T_3 is secreted by the thyroid gland itself. There are at least two peripheral enzyme systems involved in the T_4 monodeiodination: an alpha ring

Table 3. Effect of Ether and Thiopental Anesthesia on Serum Radioactive Thyroxine Levels.

Group	*Prior to Anesthesia*					*During Anesthesia*		*After Anesthesia*		
	48 hours	*36 hours*	*24 hours*	*21 hours*	*0† minutes*	*20 minutes*	*40 minutes*	*30 minutes*	*2 hours*	*24 hours*
Control (5)*	203.4 ±9.1‡	169.2 ±5.6	131.0 ±4.7	131.9 ±8.5	100	98.1 ±2.1	96.0 ±1.3	92.6 ±2.3	94.2 ±3.4	78.0 ±3.2
Ether (5)*	213.4 ±2.0	179.1 ±2.7	137.2 ±3.7	130.3 ±3.5	100	119.4 ±5.4	135.4 ±4.9	139.9 ±3.0	127.4 ±3.8	86.6 ±4.1
Thiopental (6)*	214.7 ±7.2	181.1 ±6.0	131.6 ±3.2	131.2 ±3.2	100	100.0 ±0.8	97.0 ±1.5	98.8 ±1.9	100.7 ±7.5	83.3 ±1.6

*Number of subjects; none underwent operation.
†Serum radioactivity was estimated as 100 percent.
‡± = standard error of the mean.
(From Oyama, T., Shibata, S., and Matsuki, A.: *Thyroxine distribution during ether and thiopental anesthesia in man.* Anesth. Analg. 48:1–6, 1969, with permission.)

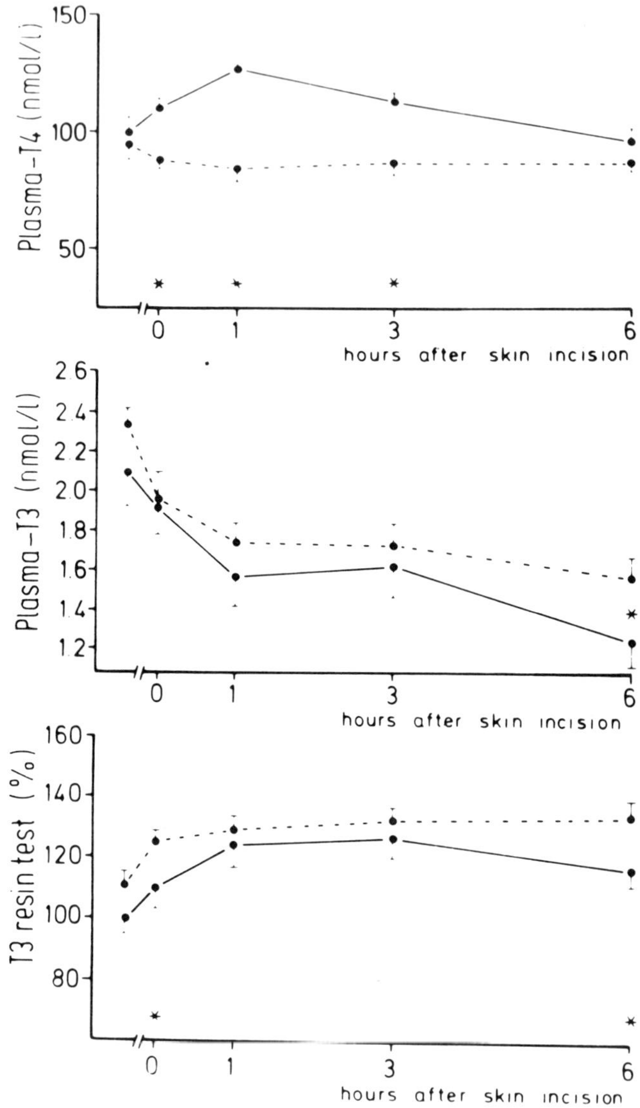

Figure 4. Changes in plasma T_4, T_3, and T_3 resin test during surgery under general anesthesia (solid line) and under epidural analgesia (broken line). (From Brandt, M. R., Kehlet, H., Skvosted, L., et al.: *Rapid decrease in plasma-triiodothyronine during surgery and epidural analgesia independent of afferent neurogenic stimuli and of cortisol.* Lancet 2:1333–1336, 1976, with permission.)

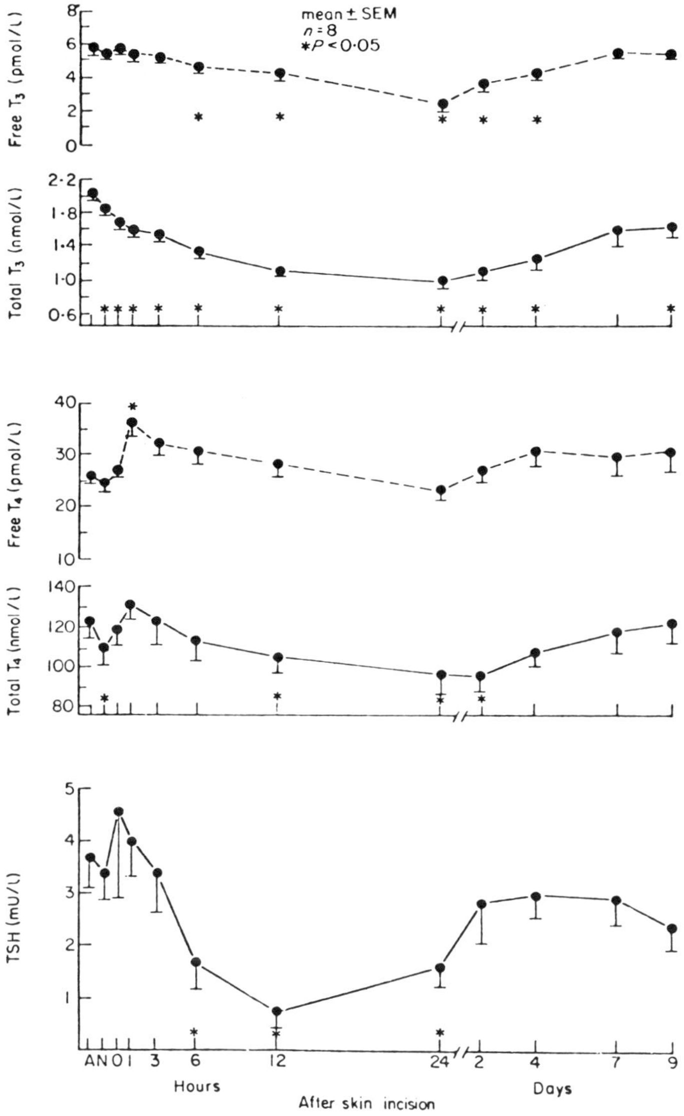

Figure 5. Changes in free and total T_3 and T_4, and TSH following uncomplicated intraabdominal surgery. (From Kehlet, H., Klauber, P. V., and Weeke, J.: *Thyrotropin, free and total triiodothyronine, and thyroxine in serum during surgery.* Clin. Endocrinol. 10:131–136, 1979, with permission.)

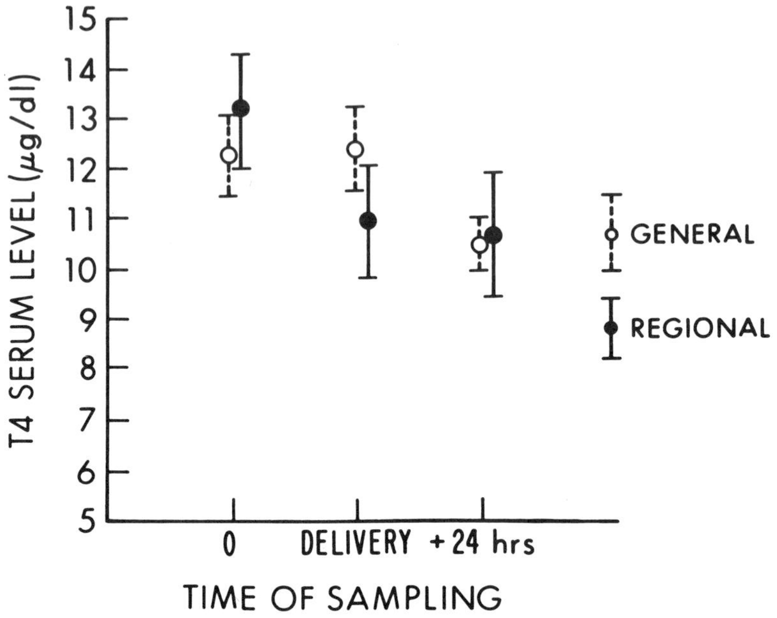

Figure 6. Serum thyroxine (T_4) concentration (mean ± SEM) in patients undergoing cesarean section under general or regional anesthesia. (From Halevy, S., Liu-Barnett, M., Ross, P. L., et al.: *Serum thyroid hormone changes in patients undergoing caesarean section under general or regional anesthesia.* Br. J. Anaesth. 50:1053–1957, 1978, with permission.)

5-deiodinase that acts on the tyrosyl ring of T_4 and produces rT_3 (Fig. 9); and a beta ring 5′-deiodinase that acts on the phenolic ring of T_4, produces T_3, and probably converts reverse T_3 to diiodothyronine (T_2). When beta ring deiodinase activity increases, T_3 blood levels increase and rT_3 serum concentration decreases. A decrease of this activity will have the opposite effects. Similar results would occur when alpha ring deiodinase activity changes.

In conclusion, the peripheral metabolism of T_4 can yield T_3 as well as rT_3.[12, 23] These theoretical considerations may be clinically very important, since an increase in rT_3 associated with a decrease in T_3 has been observed in a variety of well-documented clinical situations (Table 4).[9, 13] For example, an increase of the reverse T_3 pathway and production coincidental

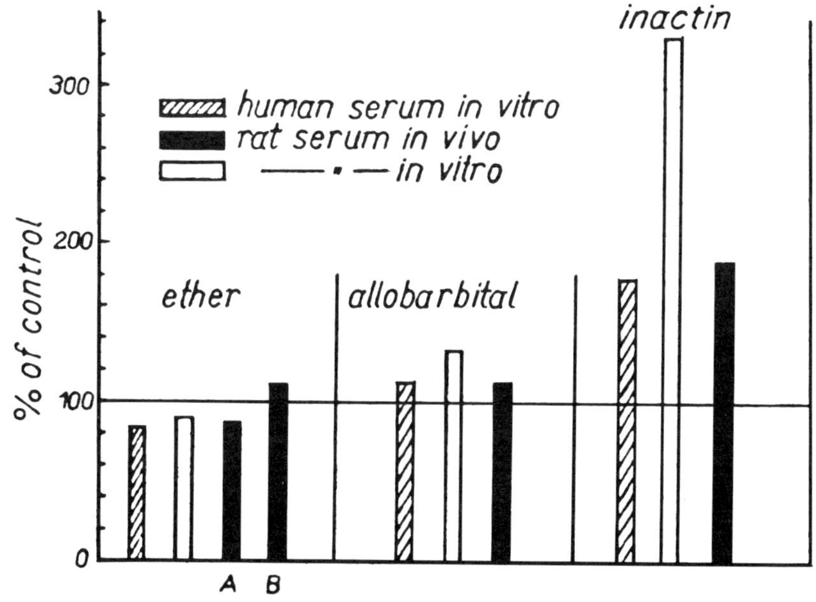

Figure 7. Free thyroxine (PFT_4) expressed in percentage of controls. *A,* light ether anesthesia; *B,* deep ether anesthesia. (From Michajlovskij, N., and Knopp, J.: *Effect of some anesthetics on the level of free thyroxine in human and rat blood sera.* Endokrinologie 62:90–94, 1973, with permission.)

with a decrease in the T_3 pathway, both resulting from thyroxine catabolism, was observed during and after surgery (Fig. 8);[8] during starvation, caloric deprivation, and fasting (Fig. 10);[50] in the newborn;[14, 23] and following the administration of synthetic glucocorticoids.[7, 15] The clinical significance of these changes is not clear at present.

Despite the fact that T_3 is the most potent active thyroid hormone,[36] only a few clinical studies of this hormone in connection with anesthesia and surgery are available. However, from the existing data (Table 2) we can conclude that triiodothyronine is decreased by surgery and most anesthetics used (Figs. 4, 5, and 11). Because of this, it seems reasonable to assume that both general and regional anesthetics may be used in cases of hyperthyroidism with elevated T_3 levels.

Both anesthesia and surgery could interfere with the peripheral metabolism of T_3. Based on the available data, it is difficult

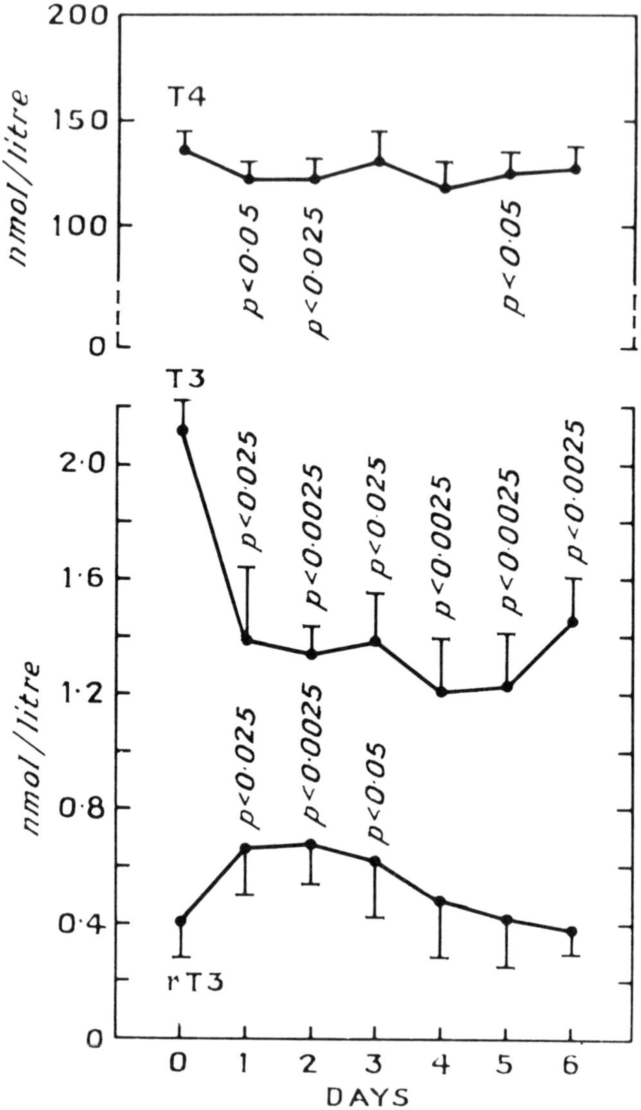

Figure 8. Serum T_4, T_3, and rT_3 concentrations in surgical patients (mean $\pm$ SEM). Initial blood sample on the day of operation (day 0) was taken before surgery. Differences from day 0 that are statistically significant are indicated. (From Burr, W. A., Griffeths, R. S., Black, E. G., et al.: *Serum triiodothyronine and reverse triiodothyronine concentrations after surgical operation.* Lancet 2:1277–1278, 1975, with permission.)

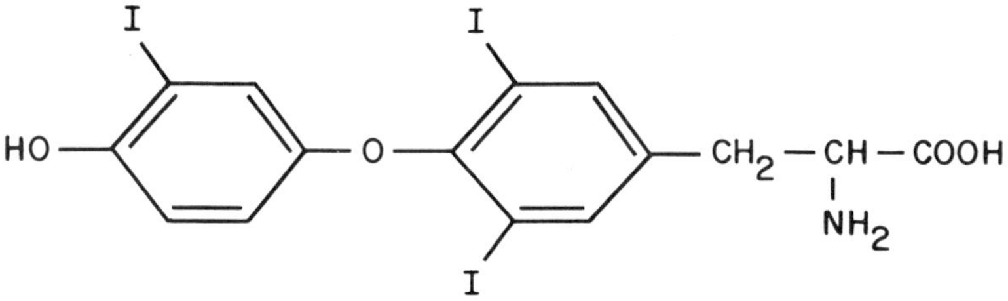

3,5,3' – Triiodothyronine (T3)

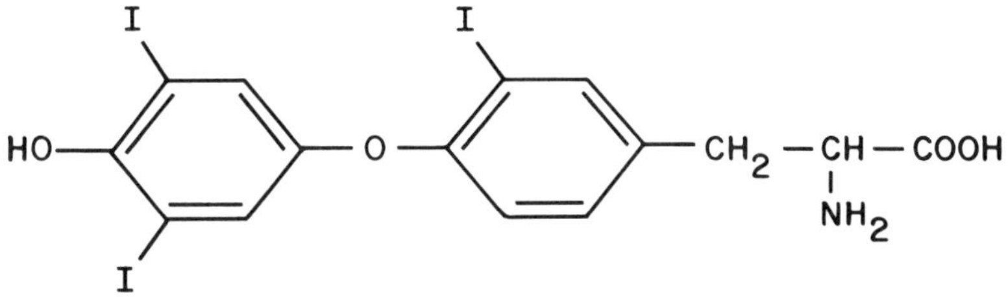

3,3',5' – Triiodothyronine (Reverse T3, rT3)

Figure 9. Molecular structure of 3,5,3′ and 3,3′,5′-triiodothyronine.

to establish which of the two factors is primarily responsible for the observed effects.

Concerning reverse T_3 and anesthesia, only two studies, including our own, are available (Table 2 and Fig. 11).[31] Therefore, no meaningful conclusions can be reached with respect to this hormonal change during anesthesia.

INFLUENCE OF THYROID HORMONES ON ANESTHESIA OR ANESTHETIC ACTION

The anesthesiologist should know if anesthesia influences normal or altered thyroid function, because anesthetics associated with an increase in thyroid hormones should not be used in cases of hyperthyroidism. Anesthetics associated with decreased thyroid function are contraindicated when this function is already depressed.

Another important aspect, insufficiently explored but which should be taken into consideration, is the effect of thyroid hormones and thyroid function on anesthetic action. New experi-

Table 4. Serum Concentrations of rT_3, T_3, and T_4 in Systemic Illnesses and Protein-Calorie Malnutrition (PCM).

Study group	rT_3 ng/100 ml	Dialyzable fraction of rT_3 (%)	Free rT_3 pg/100 ml	T_3 ng/100 ml	Dialyzable fraction of T_3 (%)	Free T_3 pg/100 ml	T_4 µg/100 ml	Dialyzable fraction of T_4 (%)	Free T_4 ng/100 ml
Normal adults	40.5†† ±2.0(27) [27–62]	0.26 ±0.012(10) [0.20–0.32]	98.1 ±10.4(10) [59–162]	118 ±8.3(16) [72–195]	0.34 ±0.01(16) [237–619]	401 ±27(16) [237–619]	8.7 ±0.33(24) [5.6–13]	0.030 ±0.002(16) [0.021–0.04]	3.1 ±0.1(16) [2.5–4.2]
Newborn cord serum	151* ±11.9(18) [95–300]	0.32* ±0.013(10) [0.27–0.41]	516* ±42.6(10) [344–711]	28.0* ±3.3(16) [<15–68]	0.18 ±0.024(5) [0.21–0.34]	121* ±18(5) [59–173]	12.7* ±0.77(18) [6.0–19]	0.028 ±0.003(5)	2.6† ±0.14(5) [2.2–2.9]
Hepatic cirrhosis	75.5* ±8.3(16) [31–140]	0.50* ±0.050(11) [0.33–0.66]	450* ±89.6(11) [102–1.085]	35.8* ±3.5(16) [<15–65]	0.53* ±0.046(11) [0.34–0.82]	181* ±30(11) [73–393]	7.4 ±0.46(16) [4.5–11]	0.054* ±0.006(11) [0.031–0.93]	3.96† ±0.30(11) [2.2–5.4]

Chronic renal failure	46.2 ±3.1(14) [30–68]	0.39*† ±0.023(5) [0.33–0.46]	207* ±27.8(5) [164–315]	60.0* ±8.3(14) [<15–125]	0.44 ±0.04(14) [0.28–0.79]	231* ±22(14) [78–386]	6.5† ±0.66(14) [2.8–10]	0.049* ±0.004(14) [0.033–0.083]	3.03 ±0.36(14) [1.8–6.3]
Acute febrile illnesses	77.4* ±7.5(11) [52–115]	0.38* ±0.043(5) [0.29–0.54]	366* ±51.2(5) [260–535]	47.3* ±13.7(11) [<15–145]	0.45* ±0.02(11) [0.30–0.60]	198*† ±45(11) [72–592]	9.2 ±0.76(11) [6.4–14]	0.047* ±0.003(11) [0.036–0.065]	4.13† ±.47(11) [2.2–8.2]
PCM baseline	53.1 ±11.8(10) [21–140]	—	—	220 ±2.9(10) [<15–41]	—	—	8.2 ±0.54(10) [6.3–11]	—	—
After feeding treatment	22.8** ±1.6(10) [15–58]	—	—	96** ±14(10) [30–188]	—	—	7.7 ±0.06(10) [5.0–12]	—	—

Normal subjects *P<0.001, *†P<0.005; †P<0.002, †P<0.05
**Baseline P<0.025
††Mean ± SE (no). (range)
(From Chopra, I. J., Chopra, U., Smith, S. R., et al.: Reciprocal changes in serum concentrations of 3,3′,5-triiodothyronine [T_3] in systemic illnesses. J. Clin. Endocrinol. Metab. 41:1043–1049, 1975, with permission.)

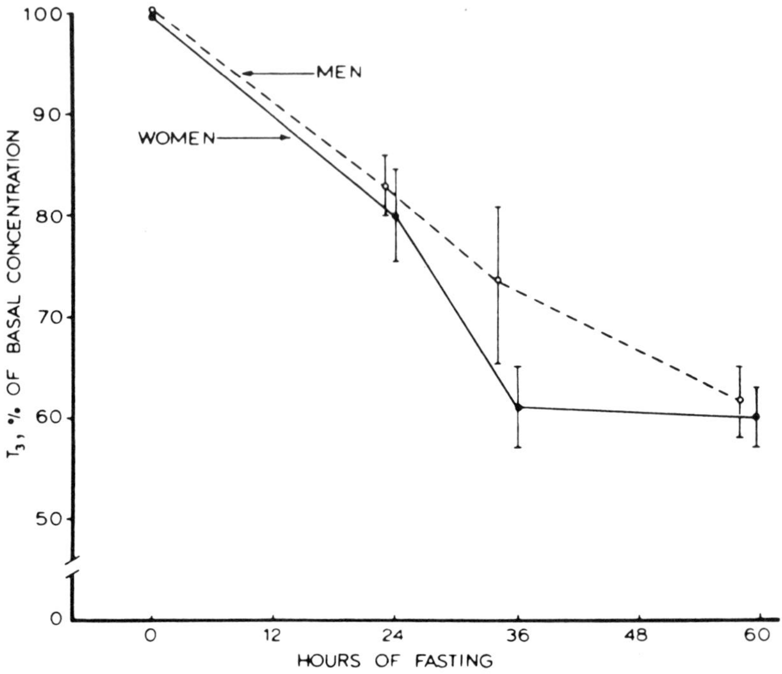

Figure 10. Percentage of changes in T_3 from basal concentration is shown during fasting for men and women. Points are $\overline{X} \pm$ SEM. (From Merimee, T. J., and Fineberg, E. S.: *Starvation-induced alterations of circulating thyroid hormone concentrations in man.* Metabolism 25:79–82, 1976, with permission.)

mental data may eventually explain clinically observed differences in response to anesthetics in individuals with thyroid problems.

Conney and Garren studied the effect of thyroxine pretreatment on hexobarbital sleeping time and liver metabolism in young rats.[16] They found that drug metabolism of hexobarbital was decreased and sleeping time was prolonged in hyperthyroid-induced rats. Pentobarbital sleeping time was also found prolonged in hyperthyroid mice. Hypothyroid mice had significantly shorter sleeping time, which was increased by epinephrine, known to potentiate thyroid hormone action.[21] This action of thyroid hormones on sleeping time has been attributed to the effect of these hormones on liver glycogen and microsomal

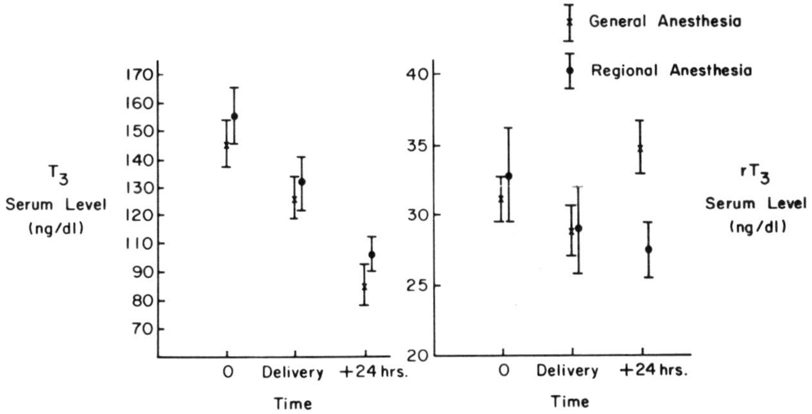

Figure 11. Serum triiodothyronine (T_3) and reverse triiodothyronine (rT_3) concentrations (mean ± SEM) in patients undergoing cesarean section under general or regional anesthesia. (Adapted from Halevy, S., Liu-Barnett, M., Ross, P. L., et al.: *Serum thyroid hormone changes in patients undergoing caesarean section under general or regional anesthesia.* Br. J. Anaesth. 50:1053–1057, 1978.)

drug metabolism. Hyperthyroidism would deplete liver glycogen and depress drug metabolism, and hypothyroidism would do the reverse. Prange and coworkers reported similar results with thiopental and pentobarbital in the hyperthyroid mouse.[70] However, pentobarbital only slightly increased sleeping time in the rat. They attributed this to a prolonged rate of removal of pentobarbital from the tissues, especially the brain. They also noted species differences in these responses. Thyroidectomy in the rat was associated with increased response to pentobarbital. Propylthyouracil treatment in mice decreased sleeping time probably by an added effect on the central nervous system, that is, less sensitivity to pentobarbital in the mouse.

The effect of thyrotropin-releasing hormone (TRH) on anesthetic action was recently presented in a number of papers. It has been shown that TRH decreases pentobarbital-induced sleeping time and hypothermia in rodents.[69] This antagonism of barbiturate anesthesia by TRH may be caused by an increase of cyclic 3′5′-adenosine monophosphate (cyclic AMP) in the hypothalamus, independent of its pituitary-thyroid action. Further experiments confirmed these data.[6] In rodents, atropine administered intracisternally antagonized the effect of TRH on pentobarbital narcosis, but not on hypothermia, suggesting a cholinergic mechanism is involved. TRH reduced sleeping time produced by thiopental, secobarbital, amobarbital, and phenobarbital, and hypothermia produced by chloral hydrate, reserpine, chloropromazine, diazepam, and phenobarbital. These studies demonstrate the action of TRH on certain functions of the brain. The sites of these actions were investigated in rats.[39] The most sensitive area in the brain was the septal region, which is a cholinergic region.

In another study using human volunteers it was found that TRH shortens normal sleep.[11] TRH appears, therefore, either as a neurotransmitter or as a modulator of synaptic transmission in the central nervous system. The practical value of these experimental and exciting data remains to be established.

CONCLUSIONS AND FUTURE OUTLOOK

It is obvious that more studies are necessary to elucidate the complex relationship between anesthesia, surgery, and thyroid function. Essential aspects, such as influence on secretion rate of thyroid hormones, direct quantitative determination of serum thyroglobulin levels, or the influence of anesthesia on thyroid hormone metabolism in pathologic thyroid conditions, remain to be explored.

Furthermore, there is a need for quantitative studies in relation to premedication, time of anesthetic administration, and depth of anesthesia. More attention should be given to age, sex, species (differences have already been noted), drug interaction, and important nutritional status of the subjects. These variables are all closely related to thyroid function and thyroid hormone metabolism. As in other areas of endocrine anesthesia, one must wait for more data before any definitive practical approach to anesthesia can be recommended.

ACKNOWLEDGMENT

The author gratefully acknowledges the editorial assistance of Mrs. Mable Pochedly of Nassau County Medical Center.

REFERENCES

1. Astwood, E. B.: *The chemical nature of compounds which inhibit the function of the thyroid gland.* J. Pharmacol. Exp. Ther. 78:79–89, 1943.
2. Astwood, E. B.: *Some observations on the use of thiobarbital as an antithyroid agent in the treatment of Graves' disease.* J. Clin. Endocrinol. 5:345–352, 1945.
3. Bernstein, G., Hasen, J., and Oppenheimer, J. H.: *Turnover of ^{131}I-thyroxine in patients subjected to surgical trauma.* J. Clin. Endocrinol. 27:741–744, 1967.
4. Brandt, M. R., Kehlet, H., Skvosted, L., et al.: *Rapid decrease in plasma-triiodothyronine during surgery and epidural analgesia independent of afferent neurogenic stimuli and of cortisol.* Lancet 2:1333–1336, 1976.
5. Brown, P. S., Clark, C. G., Crooks, J., et al.: *Thyroid and adrenocortical responses to surgical operation.* Clin. Sci. 27:447–456, 1964.
6. Breese, G. R., Cott, J. M., Cooper, B. R., et al.: *Effects of thyrotropin-releasing hormone (TRH) on the actions of pentobarbital and other centrally acting drugs.* J. Pharmacol. Exp. Ther. 193:11–22, 1975.
7. Burr, W. A., Griffiths, R. S., Black, E. G., et al.: *Serum triiodothyronine and reverse triiodothyronine concentrations after surgical operation.* Lancet 2:1277–1279, 1975.
8. Burr, W. A., Ramsden, D. B., Griffiths, R. S., et al.: *Effect of a single dose of dexamethasone on serum concentrations of thyroid hormones.* Lancet 2:58–61, 1976.
9. Cavalieri, R. R., and Rapoport, B.: *Impaired peripheral conversion of thyroxine to triiodothyronine.* Ann. Rev. Med. 28:57–65, 1977.
10. Charters, A. C., Odell, W. D., and Thompson, J. C.: *Anterior pituitary function during surgical stress and convalescence. Radio immunoassay measurement of blood TSH, LH, FSH and growth hormone.* J. Clin. Endocrinol. Metab. 29:63–71, 1969.
11. Chihara, K., Kato, Y., Maeda, K., et al.: *Effects of thyrotropin-releasing hormone on sleep and sleep-related growth hormone release in normal subjects.* J. Clin. Endocrinol. Metabl. 44:1094–1100, 1977.
12. Chopra, I. J.: *A radioimmunoassay for measurement of 3,3′,5′-triiodothyronine (reverse T3).* J. Clin. Invest. 54:583–592, 1974.
13. Chopra, I. J., Chopra, U., Smith, S. R., et al.: *Reciprocal changes in serum concentrations of 3,3′,5-triiodothyronine (T3) in systemic illnesses.* J. Clin. Endocrinol. Metab. 41:1043–1049, 1975.
14. Chopra, I. J., Sack, J., and Fisher, D. A.: "Reverse T3 in the fetus and newborn." In Fisher, D. A., and Burrow, G. N. (eds.): *Perinatal Thy-*

roid Physiology and Disease. Raven Press, New York, 1975, pp. 33–40.

15. Chopra, I. J., Williams, D. E., Orgiazzi, J., et al.: *Opposite effects of dexamethasone on serum concentrations of 3,3′,5′-triiodothyronine (reverse T3) and 3,3′5-triiodothyronine (T3).* J. Clin. Endocrinol. Metab. 41:911–920, 1975.
16. Conney, A. H., and Garren, L.: *Contrasting effects of thyroxin on zoxazolamine and hexobarbital metabolism.* Biochem. Pharmacol. 6:257–262, 1961.
17. Croxson, M. S., Hall, T. D., Kletzky, O. A., et al.: *Decreased serum thyrotropin induced by fasting.* J. Clin. Endocrinol. Metab. 45:560–568, 1977.
18. Davis, J. C., and Hipkin, L. J.: *Clinical Endocrine Pathology.* Blackwell, Oxford, 1977.
19. Ducommun, P., Sakiz, E., and Guillemin, R.: *Liability of plasma TSH levels in the rat in response to nonspecific exteroceptive stimuli.* Proc. Soc. Exp. Biol. Med. 121:921–923, 1966.
20. Ducommun, P., Vale, W., Sakiz, E., et al.: *Reversal of the inhibition of TSH secretion due to acute stress.* Endocrinology 80:953–957, 1967.
21. Ellinwood, E. H., and Prange, A. J.: *Effect of epinephrine pretreatment on pentobarbital sleeping time of mice with altered thryoid status.* Nature 201:305–306, 1964.
22. Engstrom, W. W., and Markardt, B.: *The effects of serious illness and surgical stress on the circulating thyroid hormone.* J. Clin. Endocrinol. Metab. 15:953–963, 1955.
23. Fisher, D. A.: "Thyroid function in the fetus." In Fisher, D. A., and Burrow, G. N. (eds.) *Perinatal Thyroid Physiology and Disease.* Raven Press, New York, 1975, pp. 21–32.
24. Fore, W., Kohler, P., and Wynn, J.: *Rapid redistribution of serum thyroxine during ether anesthesia.* J. Clin. Endocrinol. 26:821–830, 1966.
25. Goldenberg, I. S., Hayes, M. A., and Greene, N. M.: *Endocrine responses during operative procedures.* Ann. Surg. 150:196–201, 1959.
26. Goldenberg, I. S., Lutwak, L., Rosenbaum, P. J., et al.: *Thyroid activity during operation.* Surg. Gynecol. Obstet. 102:129–133, 1956.
27. Goldenberg, I. S., Rosenbaum, P. J., and Hayes, M. A.: *Patterns of thyroid-adrenocortical response after operation.* Ann. Surg. 142:786–797, 1955.
28. Goldenberg, I. S., Rosenbaum, P. J., White, C., et al.: *The effect of operative trauma on the utilization of thyroid hormone.* Surg. Gynecol. Obstet. 104:295–298, 1957.

29. Greene, N. M., and Goldenberg, I. S.: *The effect of anesthesia on thyroid activity in humans.* Anesthesiology 20:125–126, 1959.
30. Greer, M. A., and Solomon, D. H.: Introduction to Section 7: "Thyroid." In *Handbook of Physiology,* vol. 3. Washington, D.C., Am. Physiol. Soc., 1974, pp. 1–4.
31. Halevy, S., Liu-Barnett, M., Ross, P. L., et al.: *Serum thyroid hormone changes in patients undergoing caesarean section under general or regional anaesthesia.* Br. J. Anaesth. 50:1053–1057, 1978.
32. Harland, W. A., Horton, P. W., Strang, R., et al.: *Release of thyroxine from the liver during anaesthesia and surgery.* Br. J. Anaesth. 46:818–820, 1974.
33. Harland, W. A., Orr, J. S., and Richards, J. R.: *Increased thyroxine secretion following surgical operation.* Scott. Med. J. 17:92–97, 1972.
34. Hershman, J. M., Read, D. G., Bailey, A. L., et al.: *Effect of cold exposure on serum thyrotropin.* J. Clin. Endocrinol. 30:430–434, 1970.
35. Hydovitz, J. D.: *Effect of anesthesia and thyroid surgery on the plasma level of* PBI^{131}. J. Clin. Endocrinol. 17:76–81, 1957.
36. Ingbar, S. H., and Braverman, L. E.: *Active form of the thyroid hormone.* Ann. Rev. Med. 26:443–449, 1975.
37. Johnston, I. D. A.: *Endocrine aspects of the metabolic response to surgical operation.* Ann. R. Coll. Surg. Engl. 35:270–286, 1964.
38. Judd, S. J., Carter, J. N., and Corcoran, J. M.: *Circulating thyroid hormone concentrations and posture and venous compression.* Br. Med. J. 27 Dec.: 735–736, 1975.
39. Kalivas, P. W., and Horita, A.: *Thyrotropin-releasing hormone: central site of action in antagonism of pentobarbital narcosis.* Nature 278:461–463, 1979.
40. Kehlet, H., Klauber, P. V., and Weeke, J.: *Thyrotropin, free and total triiodothyronine, and thyroxine in serum during surgery.* Clin. Endocrinol. 10:131–136, 1979.
41. Kirby, R., Clark, F., and Johnston, I. D. A.: *The effect of surgical operation of moderate severity on thyroid function. Clin. Endocrinol. 2:89–99, 1973.*
42. *Knopp, J., and Mitro, A.: Effect of various anesthetic agents on thyroid* ^{125}*I-iodine uptake in rats.* Endokrinologie 59:405–406, 1972.
43. Kotani, M., Onaya, T., and Yamada, T.: *Acute increase of thyroid hormone secretion in response to cold and its inhibition by drugs which act on the autonomic or central nervous system.* Endocrinology 92:288–294, 1973.
44. Langer, P., Kokešová, H., and Gschwendtová, K. *Acute redistri-*

bution of thyroxine after the administration of univalent anions, salicylate, theophylline and barbiturates in rats. Acta Endocrinol. 81:516–524, 1976.

45. Larsen, P. R.: *Triiodothyronine: review of recent studies of its physiology and pathophysiology in man.* Metabolism 21:1073–1092, 1972.
46. Leppäluoto, J., Ranta, T., Lybeck, H., et al.: *Effect of TRH, and short-term exposure to experimental stress or cold on the serum immunoassayable TSH concentration in the rat.* Acta Physiol. Scand. 90:640–644, 1974.
47. Macdonald, R. G., Chapman, C., and Franklin, H.: *Thyroid-pituitary response to cardiopulmonary bypass.* Br. J. Anaesth. 48:225–230, 1976.
48. Männistö, P. T., Saarinen, A., and Ranta, T.: *Anesthetics and thyrotropin secretion in the rat.* Endocrinology 99:875–880, 1976.
49. McGinty, D. A., and Bywater, W. G.: *Antithyroid studies. I. The goitrogenic activity of some thioureas, pyrimidines and miscellaneous compounds.* J. Pharmacol. Exp. Ther. 84:342–357, 1959.
50. Merimee, T. J., and Fineberg, E. S.: *Starvation-induced alterations of circulating thyroid hormone concentrations in man.* Metabolism 25:79–82, 1976.
51. Michajlovskij, N., and Knopp, J.: *Effect of some anaesthetics on the level of free thyroxine in human and rat blood sera.* Endokrinologie 62:90–94, 1973.
52. Mitskevich, M. S.: *Glands of Internal Secretion in the Embryonic Development of Birds and Mammals.* The Academy of Sciences of U.S.S.R., Moscow, 1957, pp. 177–180.
53. Montgomery, D. A. D., and Welbourn, R. B.: *Medical and Surgical Endocrinology.* Williams & Wilkins, Baltimore, 1975.
54. Oppenheimer, J. H., Dillmann, W. H., Schwartz, H. L., et al.: *Nuclear receptors and thyroid hormone action: a progress report.* Fed. Proc. 38:2154–2161, 1979.
55. Oyama, T.: *Effects of anesthesia on thyroid function of rats.* Anesthesiology 18:719–722, 1957.
56. Oyama, T.: *Effects of di-ethyl ether anesthesia on thyroid function of rats.* Endocrinology 65:56–63, 1959.
57. Oyama, T., Latto, P., Holaday, D. A., et al.: *Effect of isoflurane anaesthesia and surgery on thyroid function in man.* Can. Anaesth. Soc. J. 22:474–477, 1975.
58. Oyama, T., Maeda, A., Jin, J., et al.: *Effect of Althesin (CT-1341) on thyroid-adrenal function in man.* Br. J. Anaesth. 47:837–840, 1975.
59. Oyama, T., and Matsuki, A.: *Serum levels of thyroxine in man during spinal anesthesia and surgery.* Anesth. Analg. 50:309–313, 1971.

60. Oyama, T., Matsuki, A., and Kudo, T.: *Effect of halothane, methoxyflurane anaesthesia and surgery on plasma thyroid-stimulating hormone (TSH) levels in man.* Anaesthesia 27:2–13, 1972.
61. Oyama, T., Matsuki A., and Kudo, T.: *Effect of ether, thiopentone anaesthesia and surgery on plasma thyroid-stimulating hormone (TSH) levels in man.* Br. J. Anaesth. 44:841–844, 1972.
62. Oyama T., Potsaid, M. J., and Slingerland, D. W.: *Effect of di-ethyl ether anesthesia on thyroid function of rats: pituitary, adrenal and thyroid relationship.* Endocrinology 65:459–464, 1959.
63. Oyama, T., Shibata, S., and Matsuki, A.; *Thyroxine distribution during ether and thiopental anesthesia in man.* Anesth. Analg. 48:1–6, 1969.
64. Oyama, T., Shibata, S., Matsuki, A., et al.: *Effect of methoxyflurane anaesthesia on thyroid function in man.* Can. Anaesth. Soc. J. 16:204–208, 1969.
65. Oyama, T., Shibata, S., Matsuki, A., et al.: *Serum endogenous thyroxine levels in man during anesthesia and surgery.* Br. J. Anaesth. 41:103–108, 1969.
66. Oyama, T., Shibata, S., Matsuki, A., et al.: *Thyroid-adrenocortical response to anesthesia in man.* Anaesthesia 24:19–27, 1969.
67. Oyama, T., Shibata, S., Matsuki, A., et al.: *Thyroxine distribution during halothane anesthesia in man.* Anesth. Analg. 48:715–719, 1969c.
68. Oyama, T., Taninguchi, K., Ishihara, H., et al.: *Effects of enflurane anaesthesia and surgery on endocrine function in man.* Br. J. Anaesth. 51:141–148, 1979.
69. Prange, A. J., Breese, G. R., Cott, J. M., et al.: *Thyrotropin releasing hormone: antagonism of pentobarbital in rodents.* Life Sci. 14:447–455, 1974.
70. Prange, A. J., Lipton, M. A., Shearin, R. B., et al.: *The influence of thyroid status on the effects and metabolism of pentobarbital and thiopental.* Biochem. Pharmacol. 15:237–248, 1966.
71. Premachandra, B. N., and Lang, S.: *Pentobarbitone-barbitone anaesthesia and thyroid function in the rat.* J. Endocrinol. 33:533–534, 1965.
72. Selenkow, H. A.: *The Normal and Abnormal Thyroid. An Approach to Diagnosis and Therapy.* Medcom Press, New York, 1973.
73. Surks, M. I., and Oppenheimer, J. H. *Postoperative changes in the concentration of thyroxine-binding prealbumin and serum free thyroxine.* J. Clin. Endocrinol. 24:794–802, 1964.
74. Utiger, R. D.: *Serum triiodothyronine in man.* Ann. Rev. Med. 25:289–302, 1974.
75. Wase, A. W., and Foster, W. C.: *Thiopental and thyroid metabolism.* Proc. Soc. Exp. Biol. Med. 91:89–91, 1956.

76. Wase, A. W., and Greenspan. *Effect of sodium 5-allyl-5-(1-methylbutyl) 2-thiobarbiturate on uptake of I^{131} by rat thyroid.* Proc. Soc. Exp. Biol. Med. 84:154–155, 1953.
77. Wase, A. W., Repplinger, E., and Foster, W. C.: *The effect of anesthetic agents on the thyroid activity of the rat.* Endocrinology 53:630–632, 1953.
78. Wilber, J. F.: *Thyrotropin releasing hormone: secretion and actions.* Ann. Rev. Med. 24:353–364, 1973.
79. Williams, R. H., Jaffe, H., and Kemp, C.: *Effect of severe stress upon thyroid function.* Am. J. Physiol. 159:291–297, 1949.

8

PERIOPERATIVE MANAGEMENT OF DIABETES MELLITUS

Jordan Miller, M.D., and
Leonard F. Walts, M.D.

More data are accumulating concerning ideal management of the insulin requirements of the diabetic patient during the operative period. Rampant hyperglycemia, provided ketosis was not present, has been espoused as the safe and effective management technique. With this method, the *bete noire* of hypoglycemia could be eliminated by overkill. New evidence questions this method, however. For example, infection is the leading cause of death in the diabetic surgical patient. Hyperglycemia inhibits polymorphonuclear cell activity and can theoretically lead to exacerbation of a septic process. Closer control of blood sugar during surgery diminishes this problem. Drs. Miller and Walts discuss various procedures of diabetes management in a practical manner.

Burnell R. Brown, Jr.

Diabetes occurs in 1 to 2 percent of the population[25] and is the most common endocrine disease. The prevalence in older people and the chronic complications experienced by the diabetic further increase the frequency of operative intervention.[1] We will divide this discussion into three major parts: rationale and management of diabetes, chronic complications of diabetes, and the decompensated diabetic patient.

RATIONALE AND MANAGEMENT

Nature of the Disease

Diabetic patients are those who have insufficient insulin secretion to meet their needs. Most cells require glucose; however, muscle, adipose, and hepatic cells require insulin for adequate glucose uptake.[12] An elevation in the fasting blood glucose is the result of inadequate insulin. When we view the disease this way we see that hyperglycemia is a symptom and not the disease. Short-term hyperglycemia in the 400 to 600 mg/dl range will not produce long-lasting problems for the diabetic. Hypoglycemia of comparable duration may produce severe and irreversible brain damage. Thus, the goal of diabetic therapy is to prevent hypoglycemia while attempting to achieve levels of blood glucose as near normal as feasible.[22] Recent evidence has indicated that diabetic patients who have a more normal blood glucose have a lower incidence of morbidity.[11, 51] The most conclusive studies have shown that good control delays the appearance of cataracts in diabetics, rapidly decreases albumin spillage by the kidney,[48] improves platelet[4] and leukocyte function, and increases red cell survival.[34] Whether long-term survival and microvascular changes can similarly be corrected with excellent control of diabetes remains controversial.[11, 22] In spite of this evidence one must clearly recognize that hypoglycemia presents a much greater acute threat to the diabetic patient than does hyperglycemia. This danger is magnified in the perioperative period since the identification of hypoglycemia is difficult under general anesthesia. Central nervous system symptoms such as confusion, coma, or convulsions will not be manifested.[29] Instead of the catecholamine-mediated responses of tachycardia and hypertension, the response to severe hypoglycemia under general anesthesia may be cardiovascular depression with bradycardia and hypotension. As such, the response of the diabetic to hypoglycemia under general anesthesia is easily mistaken for the more common causes of cardiovascular instability including blood loss, traction reflexes, and excessive depth of anesthesia. Autonomic reflexes associated with light anesthesia may also be confused for the catecholamine release caused by hypoglycemia. Therefore, to prevent hypoglycemia, keep the diabetic patient in the high normal glucose range and treat hyperglycemia less aggressively than one would in an awake patient.

Ketosis, the presence of small amounts of ketone bodies in blood and urine, is an indication that lipolysis is occurring.[12] This is not uncommon in the fasted state in normals and diabetics. However, large quantities of ketone bodies associated with acidosis is a life-threatening occurrence. Ketoacidosis is indicative of very low insulin levels, since lipolysis is inhibited by low levels of insulin.[38]

Preoperative Assessment

Evaluation of the diabetic patient must include consideration of duration, severity, and present medication of the diabetes mellitus. These will help predict the perioperative problems. Juvenile onset diabetics have lower circulating insulin levels and thus are frequently difficult to control. They vary from hypo- to hyperglycemia and develop ketoacidosis much more easily than the maturity onset diabetic who has inadequate but substantial circulating levels of insulin.[38] The juvenile onset diabetic may not tolerate starvation preoperatively because of low glycogen stores. Ketoacidosis may develop quickly in the absence of exogenous insulin in this group. On the other hand, the maturity onset diabetic frequently decreases fasting blood sugar without ketosis when starved preoperatively. A history of frequent episodes of hypoglycemia in response to insulin should alert one to the possibility of low glycogen reserves. Fasting blood glucose should be obtained as a guide to the severity of the diabetes mellitus; very high levels increase the likelihood of hyperglycemic hyperosmolar nonketotic coma.[14, 46, 54]

The hypoglycemic agent prescribed and its dose and frequency of administration will predict both peak effect and potential for hypoglycemia in the patient. Ultra long-acting insulin such as protamine zinc insulin or ultra lente or a long-acting oral hypoglycemic agent such as chlorpropramide (Diabenase)[39] may still have an effect on the morning of surgery though the last dose was given 24 hours preoperatively. Patients on these long-acting insulin preparations will require preoperative glucose administration to prevent hypoglycemia the morning of surgery.[15] Prior to induction of anesthesia the chart should be reviewed to see whether any extra insulin was given since the preoperative assessment, again to anticipate episodes of hypoglycemia. It is not uncommon for diabetics to have a positive urine glucose late in the evening or early in the morning hours and be treated with a single dose of insulin, though this was not part of the usual therapy. A morning blood glucose should be obtained prior to induction of anesthesia. This can be obtained in the operating room, if the patient is the first case of the day. Patients who come to surgery later in the day should have an early morning blood glucose drawn so as to protect against an episode of hypoglycemia[15] or hyperglycemia prior to arrival in the operating room.

Many other factors play a role in making control of diabetes more difficult in the perioperative period. There are differences in the effects of anesthetics on blood glucose even in normal patients. These relate both to differences in the effect on insulin secretion in response to changes in blood glucose as well as the effects on several other hormones that interact with insulin.[8, 12, 15, 16, 19, 20, 21, 30, 32, 45, 53] These anesthetic differences, however, are masked by the much greater though similar effect produced by the stress of surgery.[41] Numerous studies have correlated the blood glucose in diabetics with the type and duration of surgery rather than the anesthetic agent.[8, 15, 38, 53] Since anesthesia is rarely administered without surgery, we will consider the combined effect rather than separate the two.

Anesthesia and surgery raise the levels of catecholamines, glucocorticoids, and growth hormone.[1, 12, 32] In turn these hormones combine to raise the free-fatty acids and glucose in the blood and lower the utilization of glucose by insulin-dependant tissues. In contrast when surgery cures an infection by draining an abcess, glucose level may actually decline and insulin requirements may be reduced by the surgical intervention.

Methods of Management

A large number of protocols have been developed in an attempt to formulate a single mode of insulin therapy for all diabetics in the perioperative period.[6, 7, 16-18, 26, 31, 37, 38, 40-42, 49, 52] These can be categorized as follows:

1. No insulin or glucose is given on the day of surgery; insulin is given only if it is required for severe hyperglycemia and/or ketoacidosis.[9, 15]
2. A partial or whole dose of the usual intermediate-acting insulin is given subcutaneously the morning of surgery. This is covered with intravenous glucose approximately 50 grams every 8 hours until the patient tolerates oral feeding.[26, 31, 37, 41]
3. Subcutaneous regular insulin, started several days preoperatively is given and this is covered with intravenous glucose from the time the patient is made NPO. The dose of insulin is determined by urine or blood glucose.[1, 16]
4. Intravenous insulin, either single injection or continuous intravenous infusion, is given with intravenous dextrose. The dose of insulin is either predicated on the glucose infusion or titrated by frequent blood glucose measurements.[1, 17, 40, 43, 52]

While each of these regimens has advantages, it is only recently that studies have compared the risk-to-benefit ratio of each. Let us now look at each of these protocols in terms of strengths and weaknesses.

If there is no administration of insulin or glucose preoperatively, the patient is forced to rely on his own stores of glucose (glycogen) to allow for metabolic needs. The maturity onset diabetic does well with this technique, frequently decreasing blood glucose without producing ketosis, which is a sign of inadequate glucose utilization to meet metabolic needs. The juvenile diabetic, on the other hand, frequently will not tolerate even a short period of time without insulin and glucose. Patients given long-acting hypoglycemic agents may become hypoglycemic preoperatively if there is inadequate glucose to cover the continued action of these long-acting agents.[15] Most diabetics undergoing minor surgery will tolerate this form of therapy, which carries little risk of hypoglycemia. Frequent monitoring of blood glucose during major surgery and insulin therapy, when necessary, can prevent severe hyperglycemia or ketosis.[15] However, during major surgery the extra energy obtained from glucose administration and its protein sparing qualities may be useful.[1, 12]

Since the requirement of insulin is expected to vary from that required preoperatively, the insulin dose cannot be adequately predicted on the basis of preoperative experience. Intermediate-acting insulins have an onset of 4 hours and a peak effect of 8 hours. This time course usually does not correlate with glucose administration and operative intervention, which usually occur in the morning. The peak effect is in the afternoon, long after the surgical stress is over. These insulins are most active at the time of the evening meal, which is frequently not taken. Patients receiving long-term intravenous therapy need a more uniform level of insulin than provided by this therapy, so a more uniform method of insulin administration seems desirable. Further danger to these patients arises from delays in surgery, which causes hypoglycemia (in spite of glucose administration) in the early afternoon prior to the surgical stress.

While the method of intravenous insulin with intravenous glucose would seem to fit the patient better, there is no necessary relationship between the amount of glucose infused and the insulin that is needed to control hyperglycemia. Patients differ in their insulin requirements, and hour-to-hour changes can occur as the surgical stress varies.[40] Taitelman, using 2 units per hour in insulin-dependent diabetics who normally required more than 20 units of insulin per day, found hypoglycemia in 4 of 6 patients given this regimen, and only fair control of blood sugar was obtained when using 1 unit per hour in a second group of patients.[43] Woodruff has also reported more difficulty with hypoglycemia using 2 units per hour than 1 unit per hour, even though better control of blood glucose was obtained at the higher dose.[52] The method is subject to controversy. Insulin is adsorbed by the infusion bottles and I.V. tubing, resulting in unpredictability when insulin is administered with the dextrose.[1, 35, 50] Approximately 50 percent of insulin placed in an I.V. bottle or plastic container may be adsorbed to the surface, while as much as 50 percent of the remaining insulin is adsorbed to the tubing. Thus the patient receives only 25 percent of the total insulin dose. Because of this, many clinicians do not mix the insulin with the I.V. fluid, but, instead, use either a syringe pump or a pediatric administration set.[47] Thereafter, the patient receives almost all the insulin administered. With this technique a priming dose of insulin equal to the first hour's dose is given thus reducing the effect of adsorption during the first hour. When the adsorption by both the intravenous administration sets and I.V. bottles is considered, the use of 20 to 30 units of insulin per liter of glucose infused over 8 hours does administer to the patient approximately 1 unit of insulin per hour. This may well explain the success and popularity of this method. However if hypoglycemia occurs under this condition, the I.V. with insulin cannot be speeded up, as this will result in increased insulin administration; thus a second means of giving glucose must be utilized. Since the peak effect of insulin is not rapid (1 to 2 hours), a progressive decline in blood glucose is seen until a steady state is reached. If this method is chosen, frequent blood glucose analyses are required as long as the infusion is continued. In fact, continuous monitoring of glucose blood levels with Dextrostix is mandatory in the management of all diabetics. Use of bolus intravenous doses of insulin with a continuous infusion of glucose, while it produces more peaks and valleys, at least allows one to know when to look for hypoglycemia (rarely before 1 hour and usually at 2 to 3 hours).[49]

The use of subcutaneous regular insulin increases the unpredictable effect of insulin. The perioperative period is associated with great changes in subcutaneous blood flow, which may produce as much as a 100 percent change in the amount of insulin absorbed per hour. Recent studies in patients have shown that factors influencing subcutaneous blood flow, such as exercise or local heating and cooling of the skin, affect insulin absorption.[23, 24] Similarly, patients under anesthesia experience decreases in skin temperature and various anesthetics also produce changes in subcutaneous blood flow.[13, 42] Surgery will increase circulating catecholamines, decreasing blood flow to the subcutaneous tissues. Reflex vasoconstriction secondary to hemorrhage (with inadequate blood replacement), or pain, will also affect subcutaneous blood flow. Shivering with recovery from general anesthesia may well be comparable to exercise-induced increases in subcutaneous blood flow. Thus, the variability of insulin absorption may be very great. Galloway and Shuman[16] reported the case of a patient whose death may well have been attributable to hypoglycemia induced by rapid absorption of subcutaneous insulin after a period of circulatory instability. The absorption of longer-acting insulins is probably less subject to these transitory changes in blood flow to subcutaneous tissues, but prolonged changes would also compromise their absorption by the body.

To compare these protocols in insulin-dependent diabetics we have performed a randomized prospective study of 122 insulin-dependent diabetics undergoing surgery.[49] The patients were given either (1) no insulin, (2) a partial dose of long-acting insulin, or (3) intravenous regular insulin given to titrate the blood glucose. All patients had a rising blood glucose with the onset of surgery. An hour-to-hour rise in blood glucose continued intraoperatively until the patient was treated with intravenous insulin. Patients did not differ whether they were or were not given preoperative insulin. Those patients given intermediate-acting insulin in the morning and operated on by 0900 did not differ intraoperatively from those given insulin in the morning and operated on after 1300. However, the incidence of preoperative hypoglycemia increased as the onset of anesthesia and surgery was delayed, in spite of the continuous I.V. infusion of 6.25 g/hr glucose throughout the day. In contrast the patients who were given bolus insulin did not have an intraoperative rise in blood glucose (since insulin was given whenever the blood glucose increased). Thus the partial dose of insulin is inadequate to prevent hyperglycemia during the stress of the operative period, but it increased the risk of preoperative hypoglycemia. This form of therapy seems to carry the worst risk/benefit ratio. We also randomly administered one-third of the normal dose of intermediate-acting insulin subcutaneously on discharge from the recovery room and saw no difference in the postoperative glucose approximately 8 hours later. Again, this does not show that insulin is ineffective, but rather that the stresses are variable and so no single dose of insulin will be uniformly effective. The results of this study, as well as the data available in the literature, clearly indicate the need for frequent monitoring of the blood glucose in all diabetics. No single protocol can be expected to adequately manage all diabetic patients. Frequent blood glucose analysis must therefore be obtained and appropriate therapy given with intravenous insulin either as a continuous or intermittent infusion. Patients who receive insulin must be watched closely during anesthesia and in the immediate postoperative period because of the danger of hypoglycemia. Even intravenous insulin given for titration is not without pitfalls. Two patients in our study developed blood glucoses of 25 and 32 after a single injection of 10 units of regular insulin, though the blood glucose at the time of treatment was greater than 200 and the patients continued to receive a glucose infusion. Both patients showed a peak effect of insulin at *2 to 3 hours.* Thus, blood glucose must be monitored for at least 3 hours after intravenous insulin to detect hypoglycemia. Obviously those patients given a continuous infusion of insulin must have frequent glucose determinations as well.

In a similar study on 78 oral hypoglycemic controlled diabetics the response to anesthesia and surgery was quite similar to the response of insulin-dependent diabetics. No difference between the groups of patients could be observed. Patients frequently required intravenous insulin in order to prevent the blood glucose from exceeding 400 mg/dl.

MEASUREMENT OF GLUCOSE DURING OPERATION

The measurement of blood glucose in the operating room is extremely desirable. Though the simplest test for glucose is the measurement of urine sugar, the pitfalls in basing our management on urine sugar are great. The urine sugar does not always correspond to the blood glucose and never shows episodes of hypoglycemia. This is not as good a method as the measurement of blood glucose. The blood glucose of all diabetic patients should be measured every 1 to 2 hours in the operating room and in the immediate postoperative period. Because in most hospitals there is a significant delay from the time the blood specimen is obtained until the results are reported, Dextrostix[R] can be used for the measurement of blood glucose in the operating room. A drop of blood obtained from finger, ear, or vein can be applied to the Dextrostix and after 60 seconds washed off and a color comparison made to determine blood glucose. Low glucose is accurately determined and less likely to be influenced by slight changes in time of incubation; high glucose levels (>200 mg/dl) are not as dependable.[9] The strips deteriorate with time and each batch should be checked the day of surgery against a known standard, which can be obtained from most clinical laboratories. We also draw blood glucoses that are sent to the clinical laboratories for correlation with the Dextrostix measurements. The use of the Eyetone[R] meter to quantitate Dextrostix does not seem warranted. The machine requires time for calibration and standardization and most anesthesiologists cannot afford to spend this much time away from the patient.

Suggested Method of Management

All diabetics in control should be given 2 ml/kg/hr of 5 percent dextrose (approximately 100 mg/kg/hr). This is best managed by a "piggy back" infusion of the dextrose into a nondextrose-containing fluid. This assures adequate glucose for metabolic needs and, at the same time, allows for free administration of fluids for volume replacement and drug administration. A single intravenous catheter can be used. If a pressure infusion of blood is required, glucose can be administered either by infusion pump or through a second intravenous needle. Blood glucose should be measured just prior to anesthesia and then every hour. More frequent determinations may be required if insulin is given. These can be obtained by Dextrostix with periodic laboratory confirmation. No insulin is given to the diabetic preoperatively, but intravenous insulin, 1 to 2 units per hour, can be given by single injection if the blood glucose is equal to or greater than 250 mg/dl. Extra glucose is given when the blood glucose is less than 150 mg/dl in the patient treated with hypoglycemic agents. Ketosis is treated more vigorously but the same regimen is used. Many maturity onset diabetics requiring minor surgery will require no insulin at all. Care must be maintained in the postoperative period, or the intraoperative management will be to no avail.

CHRONIC COMPLICATIONS OF DIABETES

Cardiovascular Disease

Diabetics develop vascular disease at an earlier age than their nondiabetic counterparts. These patients must be evaluated for arteriosclerotic as well as microvascular complications.

In one study, 100 diabetics operated on for lesions of the lower limb, 63 percent had cardiac disease, 44 percent peripheral vascular disease, and 24 percent cerebrovascular disease.[1]

Cardiovascular complications also bring the diabetic to surgery. Aortocoronary bypass grafts are now being used and the special requirements of the diabetic must be recognized. A large glucose load in the pump prime may produce hyperosmolarity.[2] Insulin should be given, and careful evaluation of blood glucose and osmolarity is particularly useful. The expected cardiovascular instability in these patients would mandate use of intravenous rather than subcutaneous or intramuscular insulin.[16]

Since many of these patients are on β-blockers the response to insulin must be understood. Recent studies have shown that the response to insulin is normal after a small dose of propranolol or metoprolol, but that recovery from hypoglycemia is slower.[25] Severe bradycardia and an increase in diastolic pressure occurred during hypoglycemia (similar to the response under general anesthesia). This was worse with propranolol than with metoprolol. Thus the margin for error is less in diabetics on beta adrenergic receptor blockers. Anesthetics may further potentiate the effect of β-blockers, but this area has not been thoroughly investigated.

Neuropathies

Diabetics have a high incidence of neuropathy. Though this is usually sensory with pain or tingling sensations in the lower extremities, occasional patients have autonomic and motor neuropathies. Patients with autonomic or motor neuropathies may experience adverse effects under anesthesia. Decreased autonomic function may lead to orthostatic hypotension and even cardiorespiratory arrest.[33] Motor neuropathies with muscle wasting may increase the risk of hyperkalemia with succinylcholine. Careful preoperative examination can rule out significant motor neuropathy. Motor neuropathy may make the evaluation of neuromuscular blockade difficult. Azar[3] reported a patient who responded abnormally to the testing of neuromuscular blockade with a decreased twitch tension. Administration of the nondepolarizing muscle relaxant led to a diminution in twitch, which correlated well with the degree of muscle relaxation and decrease in respiratory activity, but there was neither fade nor posttetanic facilitation in this patient. The dose of muscle relaxants required for good relaxation and the dose of anticholinergic agents needed for reversal were normal. The use of a nerve stimulator must therefore be placed with care in patients with neuropathy, i.e., on uninvolved muscle. Final quantitation of block must be based on respiratory rather than on peripheral muscle function.

Regional anesthesia is useful, as it tends to prevent the response to stress and so may well be the agent of choice when surgical conditions can be met by this form of anesthesia.[21] No evidence of worsening of the neuropathy has been reported. However, whether epinephrine-containing local anesthetics should be used is more controversial. Although there are no good studies on the effect of epinephrine, *a priori* arguments for not using epinephrine-containing solutions may be made: (1) large doses of epinephrine may potentiate glucose intolerance;[12] (2) epinephrine itself will decrease blood flow to nerves bathed by the solutions. Therefore, in diabetics with decreased blood supply secondary to small vessel disease, nerve damage might be more likely with epinephrine. Alternative methods such as continuous epidural anesthesia without the use of a sympathomimetic drug might be preferable. Although not proven, it can be speculated that hypotension may be worse for the diabetic. Careful maintenance of blood volume should be preferable to use of vasoconstricting agents.

Pregnancy

The pregnant diabetic is a special problem. The well-managed diabetic will require more insulin during pregnancy and will return to prepregnant requirements rapidly after delivery.[28, 44] This must be anticipated for adequate control and to prevent postoperative maternal hypoglycemia. In the pregnant diabetic, spinal anesthesia has been shown to produce greater embarrassment of the fetus than it does in the normal parturient.[10] This is especially true if hypotension occurs. The treatment of hypotension with ephedrine is less protective in the diabetic than in the normal patient. General anesthesia with thiopental and nitrous oxide produces less fetal acidosis than does spinal anesthesia, even if hypotension does not occur. The increased incidence of both acute and early neonatal fetal distress is well documented. Neonates of diabetic mothers have a higher incidence of respiratory distress syndrome because of prematurity and other less well-understood factors.[44] A "mature" lecithin/

sphingomyelin ratio in the amniotic fluid is a less reliable indicator of lung maturation in the diabetic than in the normal. Thus, resuscitation of the neonate of the diabetic mother may need to be more vigorous and problems anticipated. Hypoglycemia is a common occurrence in these neonates and blood glucose must be monitored frequently.[28] Intravenous glucose is needed by the parturient during labor but recommendations concerning the rate of infusion are controversial.[44] Mild hyperglycemia appears to be the safest recommendation.

Renal Disease

Renal disease may be severe in the diabetic and may progress to complete renal failure. Many renal transplants are performed on diabetics and anesthesia is required for these procedures. Insulin needs may decrease since the kidney is a major organ in insulin metabolism. Some diabetics with renal failure have very prolonged durations of action of insulin and care must be taken to prevent hypoglycemia even 24 hours after the last dose. Chlorpropamide requires renal excretion and thus duration may be prolonged.[20, 39]

DECOMPENSATED DIABETIC—ASSESSMENT AND PERIOPERATIVE MANAGEMENT

Decompensated diabetic patients include those who are (1) hypoglycemic; (2) hyperglycemic with ketoacidosis; and (3) hyperglycemic, with hyperosmolar nonketotic coma.

Hypoglycemia can be readily treated with glucose infusion. It is not uncommon, since approximately 1 percent of diabetic patients in the perioperative period develop hypoglycemia secondary to over-zealous therapy with insulin.[16] These patients can be given glucose but must be watched very carefully for recurrence. The duration of insulin may be prolonged because of stresses producing a temporary reduction in absorption of subcutaneously administered insulin. Errors in insulin administration may also occur; therefore a double check of the dose is warranted. Because of the danger of central nervous system damage, it is wiser to delay surgery until the risk of recurrent hypoglycemia is past.

Patients with hyperglycemia with ketoacidosis frequently require emergency surgery.[29] Abdominal pain may well be related to ketoacidosis, especially if the bicarbonate is below 10.[5] These patients must be very carefully evaluated prior to surgical intervention. Ketoacidosis is usually accompanied by fluid loss and patients have to be rehydrated prior to surgery.[29] The ketoacidosis may be treated either by large-dose insulin or by continuous low-dose insulin infusion.[47] As the patient improves, surgery may be started prior to full recovery, if necessary. It must be remembered that the CSF pH responds to PCO_2 much more rapidly than to bicarbonate.[27] If patients with ketoacidosis are given bicarbonate to raise the blood pH, the CSF may become more acidotic, and the patient's condition worsen. A blood gas should be obtained preoperatively and the PCO_2 should be kept low in an attempt to keep the CSF pH from becoming more acidotic. Lactic acidosis must also be evaluated.[36]

Hyperglycemic hyperosmolar coma[14, 46, 54] is produced by dehydration secondary to the increases in osmolality caused by extremely high blood glucose. Characteristically, blood sugar is in the range of 1000 and the osmolality is approximately 340 to 360. These patients respond to increased hydration with a decrease in osmolality. They must be given insulin, and hypotonic solutions are frequently administered. Glucose is not usually given as the initial hydrating solution, but may be used as the blood sugar decreases with fluid and insulin therapy. Rapid shifts in fluid may produce problems[29] and the goal is restitution of osmolality below 320 mOsm/l in approximately 4 to 6 hours. The mortality of this syndrome is still high, but may be related to the fact that many of these patients are old and frail with severe pathology. Elective surgery should not be done until their condition is more stable.

REFERENCES

1. Alberti, K. G. M. M., and Thomas, D. J. B.: *The management of diabetes during surgery.* Br. J. Anaesth. 51:693, 1979.
2. Allison, S. P.: *Changes in insulin secretion during open heart surgery.* Br. J. Anaesth. 43:138, 1971.
3. Azar, I., and Turndorf, H.: *An unusual response to d-tubocurarine in a case of severe peripheral polyneuropathy.* Anesthesiology 46:371, 1977.
4. Bern, M. M.: *Platelet functions in diabetes mellitus.* Diabetes 27:342, 1978.

5. Bienia, R., and Ripoll, I.: *Diabetic ketoacidosis.* J.A.M.A. 241:510, 1979.
6. Boehm, W. F.: *Management of diabetes mellitus during surgery and acute complications.* Chicago Medicine 65:11, 1962.
7. Casey, J. H.: *Modern concepts in the management of surgical diabetic patients.* Anaesth. Intensive Care 1:144, 1972.
8. Clarke, R. S. J.: *The hyperglycaemic response to different types of surgery and anaesthesia.* Br. J. Anaesth. 42:45, 1970.
9. Crawley, B. E., and Seager, R.: *Monitoring of blood sugar during surgery.* Anaesthesia 25:73, 1970.
10. Datta, S., and Brown, W. U.: *Acid base status in diabetic mothers and their infants following general or spinal anesthesia for cesarean section.* Anesthesiology 47:272, 1977.
11. Davidson, M. B.: *The case for control in diabetes mellitus.* W. J. Med. 129:193, 1978.
12. Efendic, S., Cerasi, E., and Luft, R.: *Trauma: hormonal factors with special reference to diabetes mellitus.* Acta Anaesth. Scand Suppl. 55:107, 1974.
13. Eger, E. I., Smith, N. T., Cullen, D. J., et al.: *A comparison of the cardiovascular effects of halothane, fluroxene, ether and cyclopropane in man: a resume.* Anesthesiology 34:25, 1971.
14. Feeney, J. E.: *Delayed recovery from general anesthesia due to hyperosmolar hyperglycemic nonketotic acidosis.* Anesthesia Progress 25:45, 1978.
15. Fletcher, J., Langman, M. J. S., and Kellock, T. D.: *Effects of surgery on blood sugar levels in diabetes mellitus.* Lancet 2:52, 1965.
16. Galloway, J. A., and Shuman, C. R.: *Diabetes and surgery. A study of 667 cases.* Am. J. Med. 34:177, 1963.
17. Giesecke, A. H.: *Anesthesia in diabetes mellitus.* Anesthesiol. Rev. 2:11, 1975.
18. Giesecke, A. H., Spier, C. J., and Jenkins, M. T.: *Management of diabetes mellitus during anesthesia and surgery.* Texas State Medical Journal 60:840, 1964.
19. Greene, N. M.: *Insulin and anesthesia.* Anesthesiology 41:75, 1974.
20. Hagan, J. J., and Kendall, C. H. G.: "Insulin and oral antidiabetic drugs." In Santo, D. (ed.): Biotransformation of Local Anesthetics, Adjuvants and Adjunct Agents. Int. Anesthesiol. Clin. 13(4):127, Little, Brown, Boston, 1975.
21. Houghton, A., Hickey, J. B., Ross, S. A., et al.: *Glucose tolerance during anaesthesia and surgery, comparison of general and extradural anesthesia.* Br. J. Anaesth. 50:495, 1978.
22. Ingelfinger, F. J.: Debates on diabetes. N. Engl. J. Med. (editorial) 296:1228, 1977.
23. Koivisto, V. A., and Felig, P.: *Effects of leg exercise on insulin absorption in diabetic patients.* N. Engl. J. Med. 298:79, 1978.

24. Kolendorf, K., Bojsen, J., and Neilsen, S. L.: *Adipose tissue blood flow and insulin disappearance from subcutaneous tissue.* Clin. Pharmacol. Ther. 25:598, 1979.
25. Lager, I., Blohme, G., and Smith, U.: *Effect of cardioselective and nonselective blockade on the hypoglycaemic response in insulin-dependent diabetics.* Lancet I:458, 1979.
26. Marbel, A., and Steinke, J.: *Physiology and pharmacology in diabetes mellitus: guiding the diabetic patient through the surgical period.* Anesthesiology 24:442, 1963.
27. Marks, C. E., Goldring, R. M., Vecchione, J. J., et al.: *Cerebrospinal fluid acid-base relationships in ketoacidosis and lactic acidoses.* J. Appl. Physiol. 35:813, 1973.
28. Martin, T. R., Allan, A. C., and Stinson, D.: *Overt diabetes in pregnancy.* Am. J. Obstet. Gynecol. 133:275, 1979.
29. Maw, D. S. J.: *Emergency management of diabetes mellitus.* Anaesthesia 30:520, 1975.
30. Merin, R. G., Samuelson, P. N., and Schalch, D. S.: *Major inhalation anesthetics and carbohydrate metabolism.* Anesth. Analg. 50:625, 1971.
31. Murphy, R., and Smalley, P. E.: *Medical management of the surgical diabetic patient.* Lahey Clinic Bulletin 13:5, 1963.
32. Oyama, T.: *Anaesthesia Management of Endocrine Disease,* Springer-Verlag, New York, 1973, p. 10.
33. Page, M. McB., and Watkins, P. J.: *Cardiorespiratory arrest and diabetic autonomic neuropathy.* Lancet 1:14, 1978.
34. Peterson, C. M., Jones, R. L., Koenig, R. J., et al.: *Reversible hematologic sequelae of diabetes mellitus.* Ann. Int. Med. 86:425, 1977.
35. Petty, C., Cunningham, N. L., and Major, M. C.: *Insulin absorption by glass infusion bottles, polyvinylchloride infusion containers, and intravenous tubing.* Anesthesiology 40:400, 1974.
36. Reitan, J., Stephens, R. B., and Warpinski, M. A.: *Phenformin-induced lactic acidosis and anesthesia.* Anesthesiology 39:562, 1973.
37. Root, H. F.: *Pre-operative care of the diabetic patient.* Postgrad. Med. 40:439, 1966.
38. Rossini, A. A., and Hare, J. W.: *How to control the blood glucose level in the surgical diabetic patient.* Arch. Surg. 3:945, 1976.
39. Schen, R. J., and Khazzam, A. S.: *Post-operative hypoglycemic coma associated with chlorpropamide.* Br. J. Anaesth. 47:899, 1975.
40. Schwartz, S. S., Horwitz, D. L., Zehfus, B., et al.: *Use of a glucose-controlled insulin infusion (artificial beta cell) to control diabetes during surgery.* Diabetologia 16:157, 1979.
41. Steinke, J.: *Management of diabetes in the surgical patient.* Med. Clin. North Am. 55:939, 1971.

42. Stevens, W. C., Cromwell, T. H., Halsey, M. J., et al.: *The cardiovascular effects of a new inhalation anesthetic, forane, in human volunteers at constant arterial carbon dioxide tension.* Anesthesiology 35:8, 1971.
43. Taitelman, U., Reece, E. A., and Bessman, A. N.: *Insulin in the management of the diabetic surgical patient. Continuous intravenous infusion versus subcutaneous administration.* J.A.M.A. 237:658, 1977.
44. Thalme, B., and Edstrom, K.: *Acid-base and electrolyte balance in infants of diabetic mothers.* Acta Obstet. Gynecol. Scand. 54:129, 1975.
45. Thomas, D. J. B. and Alberti, K. G. M. M.: *The hyperglycaemic effects of Hartmann's solution in maturity-onset diabetics during surgery.* Br. J. Anaesth. 50:185, 1978.
46. Toker, P.: *Hyperosmolar hyperglycemic nonketotic coma, a cause of delayed recovery from anesthesia.* Anesthesiology 41:284, 1974.
47. Vaisrub, S.: *Low-dose intravenous infusions of insulin in diabetic coma.* J.A.M.A. 230:11, 1974.
48. Viberti, G. C., Pickup, J. C., Jarrett, R. J., et al.: *Effect of control of blood glucose on urinary excretion of albumin and* β_2 *microglobulin in insulin-dependent diabetes.* N. Engl. J. Med. 300:638, 1979.
49. Walts, L., Miller, J. D., Davidson, M., et al.: *A study of the management of diabetic patients in the perioperative period.* Abstract ASA Meeting, 1978.
50. Weisenfeld, S., Podolsky, S., Goldsmith, L., et al.: *Adsorption of insulin to infusion bottles and tubing.* Diabetes 17:766, 1968.
51. Williamson, J. R., and Kilo, C.: *New evidence that controlling hyperglycemia in diabetes is important.* Resident & Staff Physician, April 1979, p. 46.
52. Woodruff, R. E., Lewis, S. B., McLeskey, C. H., et al.: *A reliable technique for strict intra-operative glucose control in insulin-dependent diabetics.* Diabetes 26:423, 1977.
53. Wright, P. D., Henderson, K., and Johnston, I. D. A.: *Glucose utilization and insulin secretion during surgery in man.* Br. J. Surg. 61:5, 1974.
54. Wulfson, H. D., and Dalton, B.: *Hyperosmolar hyperglycemic nonketotic coma in a patient undergoing emergency cholecystectomy.* Anesthesiology 41:286, 1974.

9

THE THYROID GLAND

Dorothea E. Hellman, M.D.

Dr. Hellman is an endocrinologist with special interest in the thyroid gland and diseases of the thyroid. She presents a lucid description of physiology of thyroid function and diagnosis of disorders of the gland, followed by a concise description of several pathophysiologic aspects of thyroid disease. Of particular value to the anesthesiologist is her discussion of hypothyroidism, since little attention has been paid to this endocrinopathy in the anesthesia literature. On this same theme, Dr. Hellman discusses thyrotoxicosis facticia, a problem frequently encountered by the anesthesiologist during evening rounds and about which little has been written.

Burnell R. Brown, Jr.

SYNTHESIS, RELEASE, AND PERIPHERAL METABOLISM OF THYROID HORMONE

The function of the thyroid gland is to secrete thyroid hormone to support a normal metabolic rate. Since the major components of thyroid hormone are iodide and the amino acid tyrosine, the kinetics of iodine metabolism are critical to the storage and secretion of the thyroid hormones thyroxine (T_4) and triiodothyronine (T_3), and formation of normal quantities of thyroid hormone depends on the availability of adequate exogenous iodine.[1, 4, 11, 15, 64] The major source of iodide is food and water, although increasing quantities are now obtained via medication, diagnostic agents, and food additives. Although normal thyroid function is maintained in spite of large variation in iodine intake, iodine deficiency remains an important cause of goitrous hypothyroidism in many countries today.[4, 11, 15] In the past two decades iodine has been added to salt, water, bread, and milk in the United States so that it is now uncommon to find dietary iodine deficiency and/or iodine depletion as a cause of hypothyroidism in this country.

In the body, iodide is largely confined to the extracellular fluid.[64] Iodide is also concentrated in the salivary glands and the intraluminal fluids of the gastrointestinal tract, from which it is ultimately reabsorbed to reenter the extracellular fluid. Small quantities of iodide are lost through expired air and skin. The major clearance of iodide occurs via the thyroid gland and the kidneys.[1] Renal clearance of iodide is a function of the glomerular filtration rate and approximates 30 to 40 ml a minute in the adult, so that the majority of filtered iodide is reabsorbed by the renal tubules. Renal clearance of iodide is increased by agents that increase solute and water excretion by the kidneys. Since iodide is easily absorbed by the gastrointestinal tract, only small amounts of iodide are excreted in the stool. It would appear that urinary iodide levels parallel dietary intake, reflecting the small loss of iodide through other avenues. Chronic diarrheal states can lead to an increase in fecal loss of organic iodide, although this represents a rare cause of hypothyroidism. Iodide is excreted in both the organic and inorganic forms in breast milk, so that increased loss of iodide occurs during lactation.

The second major site for removal of iodide from the plasma

is the thyroid gland. Here, loss is not irreversible, since iodide is rapidly organified and ultimately converted to thyroxine and triiodothyronine.[64] In the thyroid gland iodotyrosines are stored in a large protein, thyroglobulin, located in the lumen of the thyroid follicle. From this protein, thyroxine is released into the capillaries surrounding the follicle by an active process located on the luminal side of the membrane of the follicle. Several steps are involved in this synthetic process. Iodide is actively transported from the extracellular fluid (ECF) into the thyroid gland, with a high gradient of thyroid/plasma iodide concentration (T/P) maintained by an active transport process. Only small amounts of iodide will diffuse back from the gland into the ECF unless this active transport process is inhibited. It is usually impossible to demonstrate this high gradient unless organification, which normally proceeds very rapidly, is inhibited by pharmacologic means. Under these circumstances, concentration ratios of several hundredfold have been reported.

The T/P iodide gradient is inversely proportional to plasma iodide concentration and, like other transport mechanisms, is an energy-requiring process.[64] Iodide transport is therefore inhibited by anoxia and by agents that inhibit oxidative phosphorylation. Thyroid stimulating hormone (TSH) is the most important physiologic stimulus that increases active transport of iodide by the gland.[18] Other anions, notably thiocyanate and pertechnetate, competitively inhibit this transport process and provide a useful test to determine defects in thyroid organic binding mechanisms.[1, 64] The activity of the gland to concentrate radioactive pertechnetate provides a valuable agent for thyroid imaging in patients with thyroid disease.[54]

Although TSH is considered the most important regulator of iodide transport, autoregulatory factors also play a role in this mechanism.[36] The most important of these is intrathyroidal iodine concentration,[7, 36, 64] since iodine uptake and its enhancement following TSH stimulation vary inversely with the glandular content of organic iodine. Rarely, hypothyroidism in man stems from a congenital defect in the iodide trapping mechanism.[53] More commonly, this mechanism is intact and responsive to TSH, with enhanced radioiodine uptake observed in patients with goitrous hypothyroidism secondary to a defect in thyroxine synthesis.[1] This topic will be handled in more detail in a later section of this chapter.

After iodine has entered the gland, it is rapidly oxidized and incorporated into tyrosines to form hormonally inactive monoiodotyrosine (MIT) and diiodotyrosine (DIT). This process is mediated by a peroxidase located in the thyroid cell. Organification is inhibited by the thionamines Propylthiouracil and Tapazole, as well as by high concentrations of intrathyroidal iodide (Wolff-Chaikoff effect).[64] Organification is exquisitely sensitive to circulating levels of TSH, markedly reduced in hypophysectomized animals, and accelerated in the presence of high TSH levels. It is uncertain how commonly genetic defects in organic binding are responsible for clinical hypothyroidism, but it is suspected that this defect is present in a large percentage of patients with lymphocytic thyroiditis.[7]

Following the formation of iodotyrosines, fusion of two molecules of DIT occurs with loss of the alanine side chain to form thyroxine (coupling reaction). The synthesis of thyroxine requires oxidative conditions and may also be mediated by a peroxidase. Nearly all agents that inhibit organic binding also inhibit coupling. Although the organic binding of iodide and coupling reaction may involve the same peroxidase in the thyroid gland, a hereditary form of goitrous hypothyroidism involving a defect in coupling only suggests that a different peroxidase may be involved in each reaction.[53]

Following synthesis of iodotyrosines, large quantities of both T_4 and T_3 are stored in the thyroid gland. It has been observed that even during prolonged iodine depletion, normal levels of T_4 persist in the plasma for many weeks.[1] Large glandular stores of active iodothyronines thus provide protection against prolonged iodine depletion and permit continued normal release of thyroxine. This storage capacity is an important and unique function of the thyroid gland and maintains a steady metabolic rate under a variety of environmental stresses.

In the gland, thyroid hormone is stored linked to the storage protein thyroglobulin. Liberation of thyroxine and triiodothyronine from thyroglobulin occurs via proteolytic cleavage of the hormones within the follicular cell. This reaction is inhibited by exogenous iodine and explains the improvement of thyrotoxicosis following treatment with iodine.[1, 59, 64] Lithium has a similar effect on hormone release and accounts for the high incidence of goitrous hypothyroidism in patients treated with this agent.[23]

Normally a small amount of thyroglobulin is released by the

gland into the general circulation, probably via lymphatics.[55] Small amounts of iodotyrosines also escape from the thyroid gland and are rapidly cleared by the kidney. However, most MIT and DIT is deiodinated in the thyroid gland, and iodide released by this reaction adds to the intrathyroidal iodide pool.[36] A deficiency of iodotyrosine dehalogenase is a rare hereditary form of goitrous hypothyroidism with consequent excessive loss of iodotyrosines in the urine.[53]

Thyroxine and triiodothyronine are bound to plasma proteins in a firm but reversible bond. Nearly all thyroxine (99.97%) is protein bound, the majority to thyroxine-binding globulin (TBG), a smaller fraction to thyroxine-binding prealbumin (TBPA).[5, 40, 57, 63] Triiodothyronine has less avidity for TBG and does not bind to TBPA, so that 50 percent of this hormone is protein bound.[40] TBG is thus the predominant protein involved in the transport of thyroxine in the plasma.[57] In view of the high affinity of T_4 for TBG, virtually all circulating thyroxine measured by current radioimmunoassay techniques is protein bound. Binding of hormone is inhibited by testosterone, salicylates, and a variety of other organic compounds less commonly used in practice. Conversely, binding of T_4 by TBG and the concentration of TBG in the plasma are increased by estrogens. Since circulating TBG is the major determinant of circulating T_4 in the plasma, any condition that alters TBG concentration will alter plasma T_4 levels. Variations of TBPA influence the concentration of T_4 far less than variations in circulating TBG.[5]

It has been impossible, until recently, to measure free T_4 in the circulation. Utilizing radioisotope techniques, it is estimated that free T_4 is approximately 0.03 percent of total T_4 with an absolute concentration in the plasma of approximately 2 ng[30] percent. Bound T_4 is considered a metabolically inert reservoir in the plasma, and free T_4 and free T_3 the active hormones that determine the metabolic rate of the animal and homeostatic mechanisms designed to defend it. Specific binding proteins for T_4 and T_3 have been found in the cell membrane, and it is likely that an exchange process occurs at the cell membrane with free T_4 or free T_3 actively transported from the plasma into the cell via binding to other intracellular proteins.[63]

In view of the high affinity of thyroxine (and to a lesser extent, triiodothyronine) for a specific plasma protein, it is clear that, until methods have been developed for the measurement of free

T_4 and free T_3, the estimate of thyroid function based on measurement of total (protein bound) circulating T_4 and T_3 is only an approximation of circulating hormone available to peripheral tissues. The clinician must recognize that a wide variety of medications will influence TBG concentration or binding affinity and that measurement of bound T_4 by currently available radioimmunoassay techniques may not accurately reflect the metabolic state of the patient.[30]

Nearly all circulating T_3 is derived from peripheral deiodination of thyroxine and not from synthesis and release of T_3 by the gland.[6] Because of differences in protein binding, the kinetics of T_3 metabolism differ markedly from those of T_4, with more rapid clearance and fractional turnover rate in the plasma.[40] It is thought that triiodothyronine and not thyroxine is the major active hormone involved in phosphorylation and other metabolic events mediated by thyroid hormone.

Under normal circumstances a constant metabolic rate is maintained by complex regulation of thyroid function.[2, 12, 14, 18, 46, 51] The thyroid gland is regulated by feedback control involving both the hypothalamus and pituitary gland. A fall in free T_4 (or free T_3) leads to a reciprocal rise in hypothalamic release of thyrotropin releasing factor (TRF) and pituitary release of TSH.[46] Increase in circulating TSH increases the secretion of thyroid hormone via stimulation of thyroidal iodide trapping, organification, the coupling reaction, and release of thyroxine from its storage protein. There exists in addition an intrinsic regulatory mechanism within the gland, permitting alterations in hormonogenesis and secretion of thyroxine independent of the pituitary.[36] Such autoregulatory mechanisms have not been found in other endocrine glands.

Many conditions affect either the feedback control mechanism or the autoregulatory capacity of the gland. Cysts, tumors, or infections in the region of the pituitary or hypothalamus lead to impairment in the release of either hypothalamic TRF or pituitary TSH and thus decrease the synthesis of thyroid hormones. However, in contrast to the feedback mechanisms involving the adrenal gland and gonads, the rise in TSH following a decrease in circulating T_4 is slow and variable. We have recently demonstrated a delay and marked variation in TSH release following total thyroidectomy, with "maximal" TSH levels observed in some patients 4 to 6 weeks after surgery (Fig. 1).[33] A similar blunted and delayed rise in TSH secretion is observed if thyroidectomized patients are withdrawn with desiccated thyroid (DT) or T_4.[22] Neither the slow metabolic clearance of l-thyroxine nor the small residual follicular tissue remaining following total thyroidectomy is sufficient to explain this slow and variable rise in circulating TSH levels. In contrast, if a thyroidectomized subject is withdrawn from physiologic replacement doses of T_3, TSH levels rise promptly and uniformly (Fig. 2).[33] A brisk and uniform response to declining plasma T_3 levels suggests that the hypothalamic-pituitary axis is more sensitive to changes in circulating T_3 than to changes in circulating T_4 or that there are several compartments for T_4 in the ECF with gradual transfer

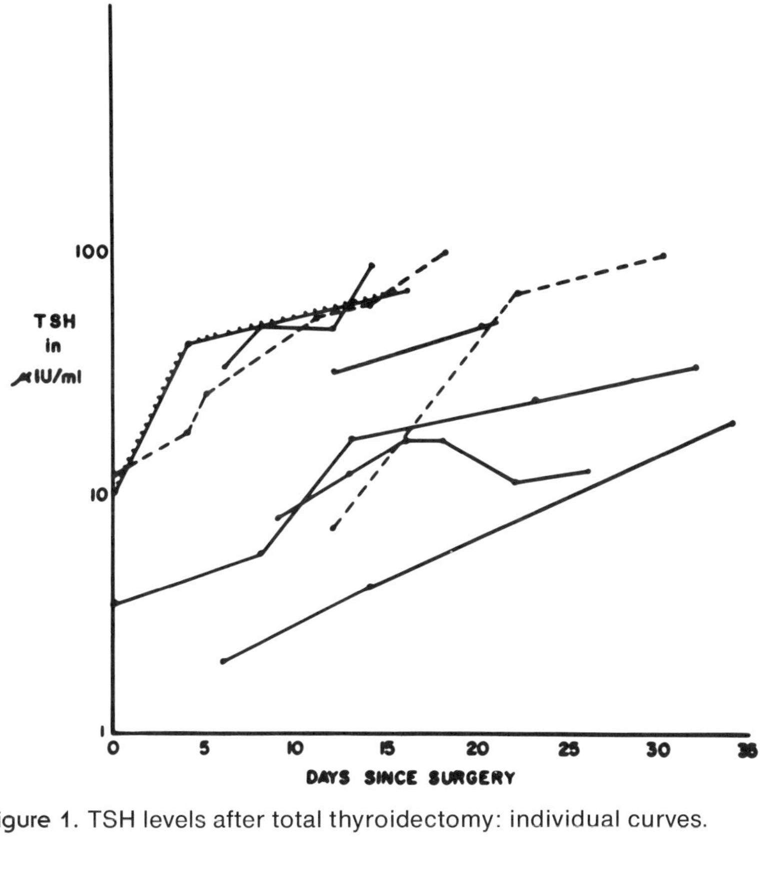

Figure 1. TSH levels after total thyroidectomy: individual curves.

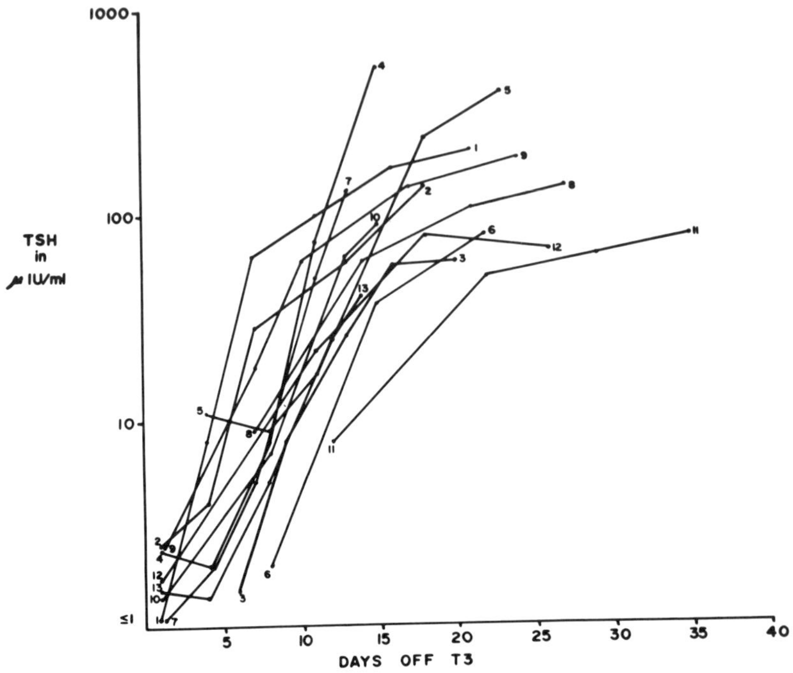

Figure 2. TSH levels after T_3 withdrawal: individual curves.

of T_4 from compartments with a slower metabolic clearance rate.

Autoregulation of thyroid function is an important factor in regulation of hormone synthesis by the thyroid gland. Intrathyroidal organic iodide concentration is an important factor in this autoregulation.[7, 36] A decrease in intrathyroidal iodine concentration enhances iodine trapping by the gland in response to TSH, while an increase in intrathyroidal iodine concentration inhibits iodine transport by the gland. Recent studies have shown that increased radioiodine uptake following acute iodine depletion antedates an increase in serum TSH concentration,[64] that TSH levels are usually normal in sporadic and nontoxic goiter associated with moderate iodine deficiency,[3] and that, following hypophysectomy, variations in iodine intake are associated with reciprocal changes in iodide trapping by the gland.[36] These observations support the hypothesis that the autoregulatory capacity of the thyroid provides a mechanism independent of the pituitary gland whereby the gland can overcome external influences that might otherwise impair its function.

FACTORS THAT INFLUENCE THYROID FUNCTION

Iodine

Small amounts of iodine administered over a short period of time appear to have little effect on accumulation of iodine by the gland or synthesis of thyroid hormone. With progressively larger doses, partial blocking of organification occurs. This decrease of organic iodine following increase of iodine intake is termed the acute Wolff-Chaikoff effect.[64] Although the mechanism of this effect is uncertain, it is known to depend on the establishment of a sufficiently high concentration of inorganic iodide in the gland. Thus, chronic administration of large amounts of iodide inhibits the secretion of thyroxine, protecting the organism from the marked increase in synthesis of thyroid hormone that would occur were the excess iodine proportionately converted to active thyroid hormone.

Although it has been recognized that chronic administration of excess iodine will decrease iodide trapping and thus decrease intrathyroidal iodine concentration, it is uncertain how effective such autoregulatory phenomena are. Concomitant with a rise in iodine intake in this country has been a marked increase in the incidence of lymphocytic thyroiditis. Many of these patients demonstrate an abnormally high radioiodine uptake.[29, 64] It is conceivable that failure of autoregulation, e.g., failure of inhibition of iodine trapping in response to high iodine intake, may lead to destruction of the gland as a consequence of high intrathyroidal iodine concentration, with lymphocytic thyroiditis either a direct consequence of such excess intrathyroidal iodine or a secondary phenomenon following release of a thyroidal globulin into the circulation and destruction of the gland by a thyroid-antithyroid immune complex.

Iodine also has a direct and rapid effect on thyroid hormone release that is more evident in patients with thyrotoxicosis than in euthyroid subjects.[64] Iodine rapidly lowers the serum T_4 concentration and acutely alleviates thyroid toxicity in hyperthyroid patients.[59] It is uncertain by what mechanism iodide decreases release of thyroxine from the gland, but such an effect is presumably independent of TSH, since it is demonstrated most readily in patients with abnormally high thyroid secretory rates. Iodine also diminishes the vascularity and hyperplasia of thyroid follicles, facilitating surgical resection of the gland. This involuting effect of iodine may reflect autoregulation of thyroid intermediary metabolism, e.g., decreased glucose utilization and energy production has been demonstrated in the rat thyroid exposed to excessive concentration of iodine.[36]

Adrenergic Nervous System

Epinephrine, norepinephrine, and tyramine induce release of ^{131}I from the thyroid gland, suggesting a direct stimulatory effect of catecholamines in the thyroid. Furthermore, the stimulatory effect of TSH on ^{131}I release from the thyroid is partly inhibited by alpha receptor antagonists. Thus, norepinephrine and epinephrine released from adrenergic nerve terminals in the thyroid may influence thyroid function by a direct effect on the thyroid follicular cell. These effects on the gland are direct, in contrast to the well-known synergistic effect of catecholamines and thyroid hormone at the tissue level.[9, 27, 38]

Sex and Sex Hormones

Thyroid disease occurs far more frequently in women than in men, and goiters are common during puberty, pregnancy, and administration of oral contraceptives. The most important effect of estrogens on thyroid economy is a consequence of their effect on the concentration and binding affinity of TBG.[43] During administration of estrogens or during pregnancy bound T_4 (and T_3) increase and free T_4 (and T_3) fall. The thyroid gland enlarges, presumably as a consequence of an increase in its synthetic and secretory activity. If the gland cannot compensate for the increased hormone requirements consequent to the rise in binding of hormone to protein, goitrous hypothyroidism follows.[26] The author has observed that women on oral contraceptives may develop goitrous hypothyroidism, presumably as a consequence of the effect of estrogens on carrier protein concentration and hormone binding affinity.

Corticosteroids

Both ACTH and carbohydrate active corticosteroids decrease radioiodine uptake, the secretion of thyroxine, thyroidal clearance, and turnover rate in man.[26] It has recently been demonstrated that these effects may be mediated via reduced serum TSH concentration.[60] The decreased secretory rate of T_4 accounts for the slight decrease in serum T_4 concentration observed in patients on pharmacologic doses of steroids and may account for the development of hypothyroidism in patients on long-term steroid therapy.

DISEASES THAT ALTER THYROID FUNCTION

Liver, Cardiac, and Renal Disease

The liver is an important site for metabolism of thyroid hormone.[57] In man, approximately one third of T_4 is cleared from the plasma via biliary excretion. The liver is also the site for synthesis of both TBG and TBPA. Consequently, liver disease may cause profound changes in serum concentrations of iodothyronines as well as in the kinetics of peripheral hormone metabolism.[57] An increase in TBG synthesis leads to a rise in serum (bound) T_4 concentration. This is more commonly seen in acute hepatic disorders such as infectious hepatitis. It has also been reported in patients with acute intermittent porphyria.[34] Conversely, diminished synthesis of TBG in patients with hepatic cirrhosis decreases serum (bound) T_4 concentration.[57] Some of the manifestations of hypermetabolism and increased catabolism in patients with severe cirrhosis of the liver may reflect failure of feedback or autoregulatory inhibition of thyroid function and high free T_4 levels following reduction in circulating TBG levels.

In patients with cardiac or renal disease, reduction in glomerular filtration rate and impaired renal iodide clearance may alter thyroid function.[5] The rise in plasma iodide consequent to a decrease in renal iodide clearance leads to a reciprocal decline in thyroidal iodine transport. Conversely, plasma iodide levels fall and thyroidal trapping of iodide increases in patients on salt restriction if accompanied by deficient iodine intake or if diuretics enhance renal iodide clearance. Patients with nephrotic syndrome may develop hypothyroidism as a consequence of large losses of organic as well as inorganic iodine in the urine. Many of these patients have a low basal metabolic rate, subnormal plasma T_4 concentration, increased lipid levels, and elevated lactic dehydrogenase and uric acid concentration in the plasma. Such alterations may reflect actual deficiency in the quantity of thyroid hormone available to the tissues, perhaps as a consequence of failure of the thyroid to compensate for excessive losses of organic and inorganic iodine in the urine. In the author's experience, many diabetic patients with nephrotic syndrome develop goitrous hypothyroidism and respond to a physiologic replacement dose of thyroxine with increased energy, reduction in fatigue, disappearance of paresthesias and muscle cramps, reduction in the size of the goiter, and reduction in cholesterol, triglycerides, LDH, and uric acid levels. More accurate assays for measurement of free T_4 are necessary in order to document impaired thyroid function in these patients.

Malnutrition and Chronic Wasting Illness

A wide variety of systemic illnesses associated with malnutrition, malabsorption, maldigestion, or increased catabolism are associated with enhanced conversion of T_3 to "reverse T_3." This presumably inert form of T_3 was first demonstrated in patients suffering from cachexia as a consequence of diminished caloric intake (anorexia nervosa). It has since been demonstrated in patients with a variety of chronic illnesses characterized by diminished caloric intake or enhanced caloric wastage. Increased conversion of active T_3 to an inactive metabolite may represent a physiologic response of the organism to starvation, reducing the metabolic rate and conserving calories. It is uncertain by what mechanism such metabolic conversion of T_3 takes place, but it appears that TSH secretion, minimal in these patients, is not directly involved.

CLINICAL DIAGNOSIS OF THYROID DISEASE

Diseases of the thyroid gland usually manifest themselves by clinical evidence of overproduction or underproduction of thyroid hormone. On occasion a goiter produces local symptoms in the neck with dysphagia or respiratory embarrassment. Large goiters may shift the trachea laterally and introduce difficulties during intubation for anesthesia. Although mild hoarseness is often a symptom of hypothyroidism, the acute development of hoarseness suggests a neoplasm in the thryoid gland with involvement of the recurrent laryngeal nerve. Ocular symptoms are described by patients with Graves disease and may be the initial complaint indicating the presence of thyroid disease.

The diagnosis of thyroid disease is established by taking a careful history supplemented by a careful physical examination. It is important that the physician recognize the subtle manifestations of thyroid disease, since marked alteration in sensitivity to anesthetic agents occurs in the presence of thyroid dysfunction and may significantly compromise the patient's intraoperative and postoperative course.

Most patients with mild hypothyroidism tolerate surgery well but may experience unnecessary and prolonged sedation from preoperative and intraoperative anesthetic agents. In the hyperthyroid patient accentuation of signs and symptoms of thyrotoxicosis during surgical stress may be life threatening. Thus, all elective surgery in the hyperthyroid patient should be postponed until treatment of hyperthyroidism has effectively decreased the secretion of thyroid hormone and restored the metabolic rate to normal.

Since the anesthesiologist is usually the last physician to examine the patient prior to surgery, he may be faced with decisions regarding management of thyroid dysfunction without the opportunity to obtain appropriate thyroid function tests. Although it is assumed that elective procedures for patients with severe thyroid dysfunction can be postponed until appropriate management is introduced, this section will deal with recognition and management of such patients if surgery is imperative, in order to minimize the risks that thyroid disease adds to the surgical and anesthetic management of such patients.

Clinical Manifestations of Thyroid Hormone Deficiency

Symptoms of hypothyroidism are usually insidious and subtle. Easy fatigability, puffiness of the face, hands, and feet, generalized aching, morning stiffness, paresthesias, muscle cramps, a dry mouth, increasing thirst, irritability and depression, somnolence, difficulty sleeping, weight gain, constipation, mild cold intolerance, reduction in mentation, and loss of recent memory are common symptoms. Women often have heavy, prolonged, and painful periods. Breast engorgement is a frequent complaint and inappropriate lactation is experienced by a small percentage of patients. Although most patients note weight gain, the appetite is often reduced. Manifestations of impaired smooth muscle function include bloating, gastric distention, and abdominal pain; skeletal muscle involvement produces weakness, aching, stiffness, and fatigue.

On physical examination the patient is puffy, with fullness of the face secondary to enlargement of the salivary glands (Fig. 3A–F). The skin is dry, the extremities cool, the pulse relatively slow. Blood pressure tends to be low in younger patients, many of whom complain of postural hypotension; older patients commonly have diastolic hypertension. Heart sounds may be muffled, cardiac output is diminished, systolic and pulse pressures are low, peripheral arterioles are constricted, and the extremities are cool and mottled. Deep tendon reflexes may be hypoactive or pseudomyotonic. The voice may be slightly hoarse or low pitched. The patient is depressed, lethargic, withdrawn, and less animated. The abdomen may be bloated with palpable loops of bowel impacted with stool. The breasts are frequently engorged and tender with clear fluid occasionally expressed from both nipples. The electrocardiogram frequently reveals low voltage or abnormalities in repolarization. Studies of cardiovascular function demonstrate low cardiac output and depressed myocardial contractility.[8, 25] The electroencephalogram may show diffuse and nonspecific slowing of alpha waves. Hypoventilation may be severe and lead to hypoxia and hypercapnia.[62] Hearing loss of the perceptive type and tinnitus are common.

Neurologic symptoms involve the entire nervous system.[20, 21, 31, 48, 50] Many patients describe irritability, depression, and emotional lability. There is often slowing of intellectual function; loss of initiative, motivation, and drive; somnolence; and memory defects. Movements may be slow and clumsy. Patients often experience dizziness and slight ataxia, especially with initiation of movement. Dementia, paranoia, depression, and a psychotic delusional state with increasing confusion and coma are complications of prolonged and untreated hypothyroidism, especially in elderly patients.

Muscle mass may be slightly increased, and the muscles may be slightly firmer than normal.[45] Rarely, marked increase in mass and tone of muscle accompanied by decrease in muscle strength may be the predominant manifestation of hypothyroidism (Hoffman's syndrome). On histologic examination, the muscles are pale and swollen with loss of normal striation and separation of muscle fibers by mucinous deposits.

Renal blood flow and glomerular filtration rate are generally decreased with increased tubular reabsorption of sodium and water, accounting for the increase in total body sodium and water.[16] Occasionally there is coexistent impairment of free water clearance and hyponatremia in the presence of an increase in total body sodium.[17] Disturbances in potassium excretion are rare. Urinary excretion of calcium and bone formation and resorption are decreased. Rarely, an increase in bone mass is observed radiographically. Serum calcium levels may be depressed or slightly elevated. Bone pain is uncommon, but aching and stiffness of joints is commonly described and joint effusions occasionally observed.

Thyroid hormone is essential for the development of the nervous system.[20, 21, 50] If thyroid hormone deficiency is not corrected in the neonate, irreversible brain damage results, with severe mental and motor retardation, visual impairment, and hearing loss.[11] Since there is little placental transfer of thyroxine, neonatal hypothyroidism is the consequence of failure of the thyroid gland to develop normally during gestation. The infant demonstrates abnormal ossification of facial bones, retardation of bone age, severe hypotonia of skeletal muscles, enlargement of the tongue, reduced reflexes, poor responsiveness, lethargy, and failure to thrive.[11] Feeding problems, constipation, a hoarse cry, somnolence, severe lethargy, protuberance of the abdomen, dry skin, poor growth of hair and nails, delayed eruption of deciduous teeth, delay in reaching normal milestones of development, and an umbilical hernia are all early and important clinical signs of neonatal hypothyroidism. Linear growth is impaired, resulting in dwarfism with the limbs disproportionately short in relationship to the trunk. Closure of the fontanelles is

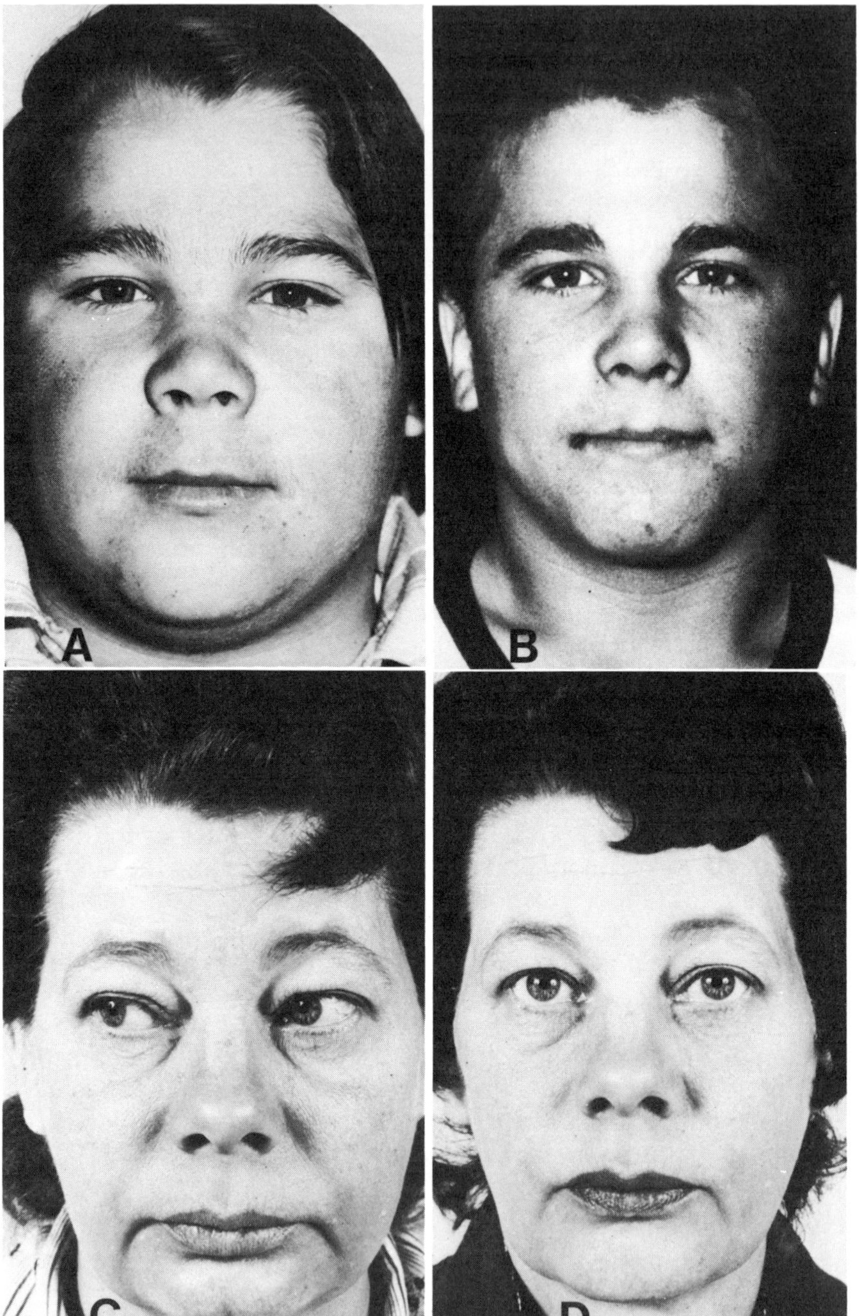
A
B
C
D

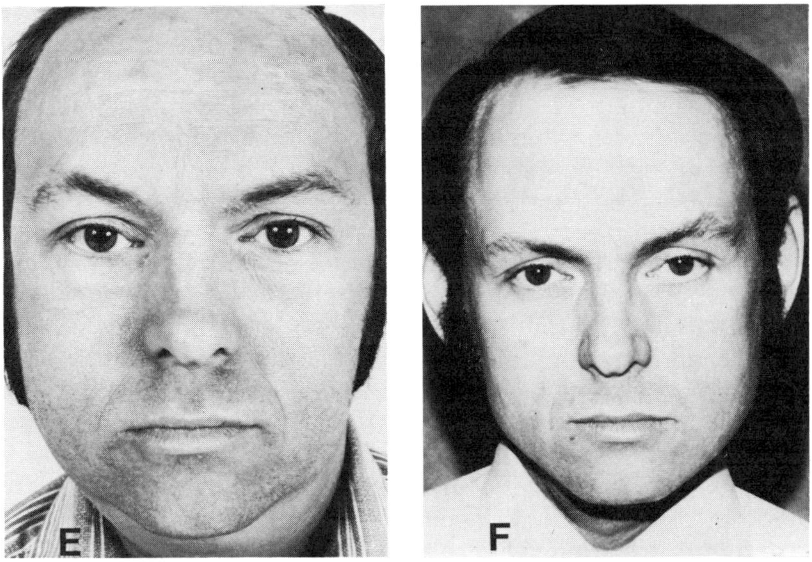

Figure 3. *A,* Hypothyroidism in a 17-year-old boy who had growth arrest at age 13, with advanced bone age and short stature. *B,* Same patient 6 weeks after replacement therapy with l-thyroxine 150 mcg daily. *C,* This woman complained of fatigue, lethargy, muscle cramps, headaches, and paresthesias, and had a cholesterol of 876 mg percent and triglycerides of 2000 mg percent. *D,* The same patient 6 weeks after thyroxine therapy had a cholesterol of 240 mg percent and triglycerides of 286 mg percent. *E,* A 31-year-old, athyreotic (follicular carcinoma thyroid) male before thyroxine therapy. *F,* The same patient after thyroxine therapy.

delayed, leading to a head that is large in relation to the rest of the body. Maldevelopment of the femoral epiphyses results in a waddling gait.[61] The teeth are malformed with delayed dentition and frequent development of caries.

When hypothyroidism develops later in childhood the clinical manifestations are less severe, developmental retardation is milder, and growth may be normal or nearly normal with residual disproportionately short extremities. Linear growth tends to be disproportionately slow in comparison to weight gain. Puberty may be delayed or premature in onset. Intellectual performance is generally poor, but severe mental retardation is less common. Epiphyseal union is delayed, resulting in retardation of bone age.[61]

Early treatment of the neonatal cretin is critical if mental retardation is to be avoided. A delay of even a few months in replacement therapy results in permanent and very severe retardation.[11] Delayed recognition and treatment also affect growth and bone maturation. Replacement thyroxine therapy reverses some of the neurologic and metabolic abnormalities of childhood hypothyroidism, although "catch up" growth rarely occurs, so that short stature is a common consequence of unrecognized and untreated hypothyroidism in childhood. However, dramatic improvement may occur in some children following thyroid hormone therapy if such therapy is instituted promptly once the diagnosis is made.

In the adult, the onset of hypothyroidism is usually so insidious that classical clinical manifestations of this disorder may take months or even years to appear. They frequently go unnoticed by physicians well acquainted with the patient, and symptoms of progressive fatigue, lethargy, depression, increased confusion, and slowed mentation are often ascribed to a primary psychiatric disorder. This slow development of hypothyroidism secondary to atrophy or chronic inflammation of the gland contrasts with the more rapid development of hypothyroidism following thyroidectomy, ablation of the thyroid gland with radioactive iodine, or withdrawal of replacement thyroid therapy in the athyreotic patient.[22, 33]

A decrease in thyroid hormone concentration in the plasma is common in all patients with hypothyroidism. In preceding years, the standard test to estimate thyroid function was measurement of the basal metabolic rate. Because this test was time consuming, cumbersome, affected by a variety of physiologic and environmental factors, and demonstrated wide overlap between normal and abnormal subjects, it has been replaced by assays that measure circulating T_4 and T_3 in the plasma.

Older methods for measuring circulating iodothyronines (PBI and BEI) were influenced by organic and inorganic iodine intake. Consequently, newer assays measured thyroxine by competitive protein binding (Murphy-Pattee). This assay gave relatively reliable results and generally supported the clinical impression of thyroid dysfunction.

Radioimmunoassay (RIA) techniques have recently been introduced for measuring T_4 and T_3 in the plasma (and the thyroid gland[10]). This method is exquisitely sensitive, measuring all circulating iodothyronines without the error introduced by losses of hormone during the older competitive protein-binding assay. Consequently, many hypothyroid patients have T_4 levels by RIA in the "euthyroid range" as reported by most commercial laboratories.[30] Restandardization of the curve for euthyroid subjects and patients with thyroid disease will be necessary before the T_4 by RIA can be used to confirm a clinical diagnosis of hypothyroidism.

Initial studies suggested that TSH secretion would rise promptly in response to a fall in either the free T_4 or free T_3 level in patients with primary hypothyroidism, and that TSH concentration in the plasma would be a sensitive assay for the laboratory diagnosis of primary hypothyroidism.[12] However, recent clinical studies in our laboratory (Hellman, D., and Nicoloff, J., unpublished data) suggest that a significant number of patients with primary hypothyroidism have TSH levels, if performed by commercial laboratories, similar to TSH levels observed in euthyroid subjects.[30] It is possible that more sensitive TSH assays would discriminate between euthyroid and hypothyroid subjects, but such assays are at present not available to the practicing physician.

A diagnosis of hypothyroidism can be established in patients by documenting enhanced TSH response to intravenous administration of TRF.[51] Unfortunately, this test is cumbersome, expensive for the patient, and often impractical for the physician to perform in an office or hospital practice. Furthermore, patients with primary hypothalamic or pituitary disease will have low TSH levels and diminished TSH response to TRF as a consequence of gradual atrophy of thyrotropin-secreting cells. Thus, elevated TSH levels are helpful to confirm the diagnosis of primary hypothyroidism while normal TSH levels do not exclude the diagnosis of either primary or secondary hypothyroidism.

In euthyroid subjects, radioiodine uptakes are reciprocally reduced with higher iodine intake.[42, 64] Furthermore, patients with defects in oxidation or organification of iodine will display high radioiodine uptake, presumably as a consequence of normal feedback or autoregulatory function of the gland.[53] As a result of changes in iodine intake, measurement of ^{131}I uptake by the gland is no longer useful to confirm the diagnosis of either primary or secondary hypothyroidism.

The physician is thus faced with a plethora of laboratory tests of thyroid function, none of which are currently reliable for confirming a diagnosis of hypothyroidism. A relatively new assay for measurement of free thyroxine has recently been developed.* Preliminary studies of this assay in hypothyroid patients and euthyroid subjects or patients on physiologic replacement doses of thyroid hormone suggest that this assay is reliable for the diagnosis of hypothyroidism.[30] Free T_4 is less than 1.7 ng percent in the majority of hypothyroid patients with a mean of 1.26 ng percent. The mean free T_4 of euthyroid subjects and patients on a physiologic replacement dose of l-thyroxine is 2.3 ng percent with a range of 1.5 to 3.5 ng percent, with overlap of values in the lower range in the three patient groups (Fig. 4).† This assay in our preliminary study of 147 subjects reflected more accurately the metabolic state of the subject than the (bound) T_4 by RIA or TSH levels. When the free T_4 assay becomes commercially available, it may be a more accurate test to estimate the amount of circulating thyroid hormone available to peripheral tissues.

In addition to the signs and symptoms elicited by careful history and physical examination, additional laboratory data may support the diagnosis of hypothyroidism. Many patients have elevated plasma cholesterol, triglycerides, and lactic dehydrogenase levels. Mild anemia is seen in occasional patients. As noted earlier, the electrocardiogram may show nonspecific abnormalities in repolarization or low voltage. Finally, the electroencephalogram often shows diffuse nonspecific slowing of alpha waves.

A clinical trial of a physiologic replacement dose of l-thyroxine (2.24 mcg/kg body weight/day) for 3 to 4 months can be used to confirm the diagnosis of suspected hypothyroidism.[12] Euthyroid patients demonstrate no response to such therapy, whereas hypothyroid patients characteristically experience a slow resolution of symptoms and slow disappearance of the clinical stig-

---

*The Diagnostic Laboratory (A Damon Laboratory), Boston, Massachusetts.

†This study was supported by a research grant from The Diagnostic Laboratory (A Damon Laboratory), Tucson, Arizona.

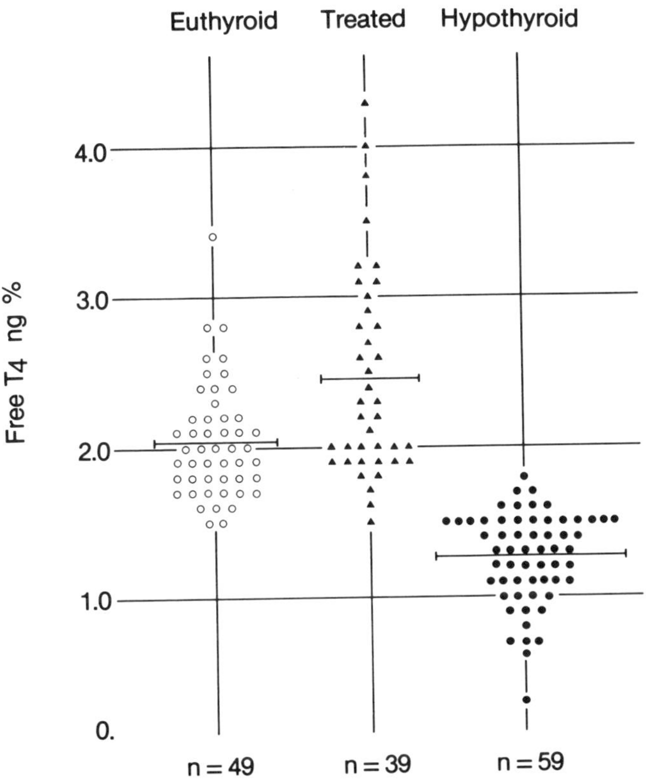

Figure 4. Free T_4 in euthyroid, treated hypothyroid, and hypothyroid subjects. The difference in mean T_4 between hypothyroid and normal or treated subjects is significant with a $p<0.00005$.

mata of hypothyroidism. Coincident with resolution of clinical signs and symptoms, cholesterol, triglycerides, and LDH levels, when abnormal, frequently decline to normal, and the ECG and EEG return to normal, tending to substantiate the diagnosis. Such replacement therapy utilized as a clinical trial is usually well tolerated by the patient and superior to dismissal of the diagnosis in a symptomatic patient. In short, at a time when laboratory tests have become difficult to interpret in the hypothyroid patient, treatment of the patient is superior to treatment of confusing laboratory tests.

Replacement therapy in most healthy adults can start with a

full replacement dose of l-thyroxine. The usual replacement dose of l-thyroxine is 100 to 200 mcg/day. This dose should be modified initially every 2 to 3 months, depending primarily on clinical response. Such titration is not facilitated by obtaining repeat analyses of plasma T_4, T_3, or TSH unless the physician is uncertain about the clinical response or unless low circulating TSH levels are considered desirable, as in patients with thyroid cancer.[19, 22, 33]

In a patient with long-standing and severe hypothyroidism or coexisting coronary artery disease, 25 to 50 mcg of thyroxine daily should be administered initially. This dose should be increased by 25-mcg increments every 7 to 10 days in order to prevent excessive irritability, excitation, nervousness, palpitations, or increasing angina. The dose of thyroid hormone in children is best calculated utilizing body weight. Postmenopausal females frequently have a lower requirement for thyroxine (100 mcg or less daily), presumably because of lowered circulating estrogen levels. Patients should be questioned frequently about any side effects from thyroid hormone, such as headaches, palpitations, breathlessness, shakiness, nervousness, or difficulty sleeping. On occasion, increasing weakness, exhaustion, and unexplained weight loss are the only manifestations of excess thyroid hormone administration, especially in elderly patients.

Myxedema Coma

Myxedema coma is a complication of severe and long-standing hypothyroidism usually precipitated by stress and accompanied by profound physiologic changes secondary to marked depletion of tissue thyroid hormone stores.[48] Myxedema coma occurs more commonly in elderly patients during infection, respiratory failure, trauma, or surgery.

The treatment of myxedema coma consists of the rapid administration of relatively large doses of thyroid hormone, given orally or parenterally.[35] Thyroxine 100 mcg every 8 hours is generally effective in reversing the symptoms and signs of myxedema coma and avoids the tachyarrhythmias that may occur with larger doses. Although triiodothyronine has been recommended as initial treatment because of its more rapid onset of action, adequate doses of thyroxine appear to be equally effective in correcting the severe hypometabolic state. Adrenal function is generally adequate in patients with myxedema coma, but hydrocortisone should be administered intravenously until normal adrenal function can be documented. Intravenous solutions containing isotonic saline with glucose are preferable to hypotonic saline in order to avoid a dilutional syndrome.[16] Assisted ventilation and controlled oxygen administration may be necessary in patients with depressed respiratory function and pulmonary disease.[62] External warming should be avoided in order not to increase the metabolic rate. Careful attention to nursing details with frequent turning, assisted respiration, coughing, and attention to bowel and bladder function is necessary in order to avoid pulmonary infection, hypercapnia, anoxia, fecal impaction, and urinary retention. All patients on large doses of oral or intramuscular thyroxine require continuous cardiac monitoring in order to detect atrial or ventricular irritability.[27] Such irritability necessitates temporary reduction in thyroxine dosage.

Utilizing these measures, the improvement in survival of patients with myxedema coma has been dramatic, exceeding 90 percent in most medical centers. Reversal of coma will occur in 24 to 48 hours; mentation improves steadily but may not return to normal for several weeks; body temperature, heart rate, and blood pressure usually return to normal in 7 to 10 days. Fluid retention clears more slowly over several weeks. After the initial treatment of myxedema coma and following adequate reversal of the signs of severe hypothyroidism, a physiologic replacement dose of thyroxine should be established and maintained indefinitely.[12]

Myxedema coma and severe untreated hypothyroidism are conditions that contraindicate all elective surgery. Correction of long-standing hypothyroidism often requires several weeks of thyroxine replacement therapy. If emergency surgery is necessary, a period of at least 48 hours should be utilized to initiate repletion of tissue thyroxine stores. Patients with partially treated hypothyroidism undergoing surgery exhibit slow recovery from inhalation anesthesia with prolonged sedation, poor bowel and bladder function, and marked alteration in the level of consciousness.[20, 21, 50] When emergency surgery is required in the hypothyroid patient, parenteral thyroxine should be administered prior to, during, and following surgery, until medication can be safely administered by mouth. A physiologic replacement dose of thyroxine (150 mcg daily) is adequate for most hypothyroid patients; the dose of thyroxine may have to be increased temporarily (100 mcg every 8 hours) in the patient with severe hypothyroidism in order to minimize the risk of profound CNS depression following anesthesia, to enhance wound healing, and to facilitate recovery following surgical stress. The dose of thyroxine should be decreased to a physiologic replacement dose as soon as neurologic recovery from anesthesia has occurred and the patient is alert, oriented, and able to cooperate with the personnel involved in his medical care.

Clinical Manifestations of Excess Thyroid Hormone

HYPERTHYROIDISM

Clinical signs and symptoms in the hyperthyroid patient are the consequence of tissue exposure to excessive concentration of thyroid hormone. Symptoms include increased nervousness, weight loss with or without a change in appetite, tremulousness, palpitations, headaches, change in bowel habits, increased thirst and urination, muscle weakness, easy fatigability and exhaustion, difficulty sleeping, heat intolerance, and increased sweating.[24] On clinical examination skin temperature is usually elevated, there is a fine tremor of the extended hands or a coarser tremor and jerking of the trunk. The pulse rate and pulse pressure are elevated; the heart is hyperkinetic;[27, 38] reflexes are brisk. The patient is restless, with rapid and jerky movements, and exhibits evidence of proximal muscle weakness (more common in males than females), recent weight loss, emotional lability, irritability, and depression.[24, 31]

A stare and lid lag are ocular manifestations of increased sympathetic tone to the muscle inserting in the eyelid (Müller's muscle) (Fig. 5*A*). Exophthalmus is caused by swelling of the extraocular muscles, which inhibits lymphatic drainage from the orbit. This produces swelling of the orbital contents with increased intraorbital pressure, pain, proptosis, injection of conjunctivae, tearing, a sensation of a foreign body in the eye, diplopia, and, rarely, loss of visual acuity owing to pressure on the optic nerve or its vascular supply. Proptosis, periorbital puffiness, chemosis, and discordant extraocular muscles when the eyes focus on a moving object are evident on clinical examination (Fig. 5*C–F*). Exophthalmus is often symptomatic before objective evidence of the disease develops and should be noted carefully by the physician, since this complication of thyrotoxicosis is often aggravated by surgical stress.

Long-standing thyrotoxicosis is associated with increased turnover and renal clearance of calcium and phosphorus. Radiographically there is osteopenia of the skeleton. On histologic examination, mixed metabolic bone disease is evident with areas of osteomalacia (decreased bone mineralization), osteoporosis (decreased bone matrix), and osteitis fibrosis cystica (enhanced bone turnover).

Mild anemia and relative lymphocytosis are common findings. Approximately 20 percent of patients will have a reduction in total white count, neutropenia, lymphocytosis, a palpable spleen, and hyperplasia of lymphatic tissue. It is uncertain whether these changes are manifestations of an autoimmune disorder or are a direct effect of thyroid hormone on bone marrow and lymphatic tissue. Severe and long-standing thyrotoxicosis may be associated with relative adrenal hypofunction secondary to accelerated metabolism of cortisol and its metabolites.[49] Although most studies of adrenal function are normal in thyrotoxic patients, response to prolonged ACTH stimulation is often subnormal, suggesting reduction in adrenal reserve. Relative adrenal insufficiency may be a hazard in these patients during surgical stress.

Graves disease is a multisystem disease characterized by diffuse toxic goiter, infiltrative ophthalmopathy, and occasionally infiltrative dermopathy. This complex disorder is occasionally associated with other autoimmune disorders such as rheumatoid arthritis, bronchial asthma, pernicious anemia, diabetes mellitus, and myasthenia gravis. A number of circulating immunoglobulins have been found in the plasma of some but not all patients with Graves disease and may help in establishing the diagnosis.[37] An abnormal immune complex, following release of thyroglobulin (TG) from the gland into the general circulation and formation of TG-anti-TG antibodies, may be responsible for the associated exophthalmus, with passage of the TG-anti-TG complex via lymphatics to the orbit and fixation of this immune complex to the external membrane of the extraocular muscles.[39]

Laboratory tests to confirm the diagnosis of thyrotoxicosis in-

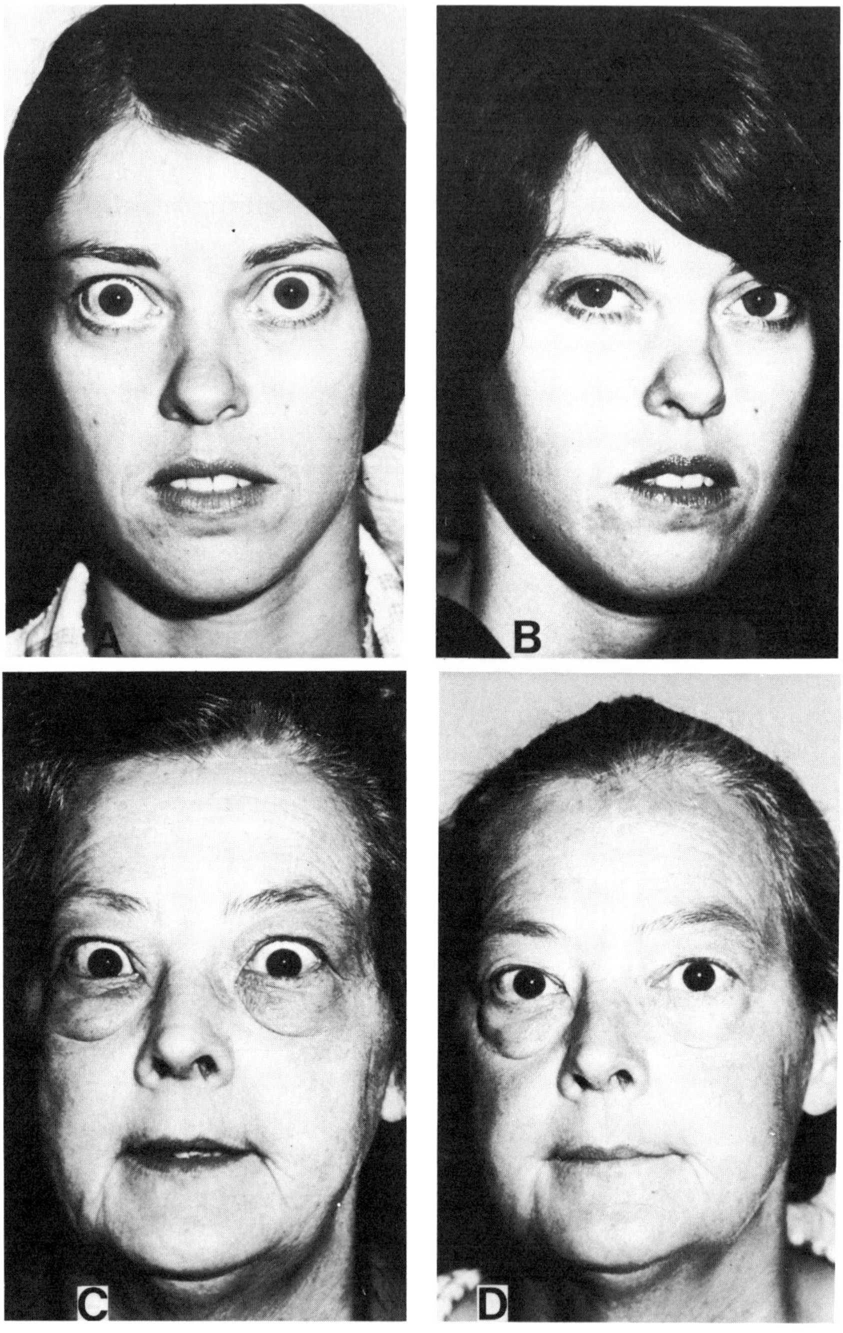
A
B
C
D

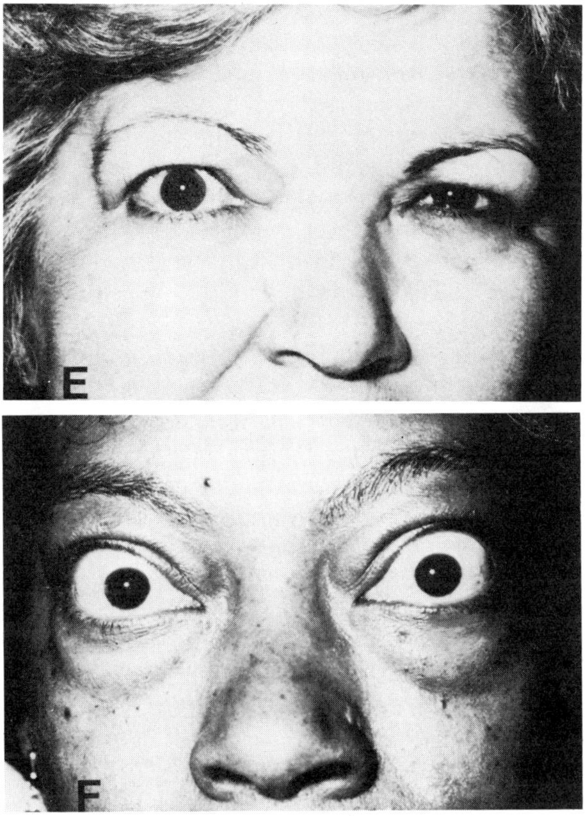

Figure 5. Graves disease. *A,* A woman with thyrotoxicosis and mild exophthalmos. *B,* The same patient 6 weeks after radioiodine therapy. *C,* A woman with severe hyperthyroidism and exophthalmos. *D,* The same patient 2 years after radioiodine therapy. *E,* A woman with exophthalmos and mild hyperthyroidism. *F,* A woman with severe exophthalmos following an ablative dose of radioactive iodine. (Note severe orbital edema, chemosis, and asymmetrical involvement of patients with exophthalmos in *C, E,* and *F.*)

clude documenting elevated T_4 and T_3 concentration in the plasma, an increase in free thyroxine concentration, abnormally high radioiodine uptake, increase in technetium uptake, and elevation of basal metabolic rate. Supporting laboratory evidence includes relative lymphocytosis, elevation of fasting blood sugar, relative carbohydrate intolerance, elevation of alkaline phosphatase, elevation of serum and urinary calcium, abnormal liver function tests, and radiographic evidence of osteopenia. Computerized axial tomography of the orbit may demonstrate swelling of extraocular muscles indicative of ophthalmopathy. In the majority of hyperthyroid patients there is absence of homeostatic control of thyroid function so that pharmacologic doses of thyroid hormone fail to inhibit iodine trapping by the gland.[58] In most patients the diagnosis of thyrotoxicosis is evident without demonstrating absence of thyroid suppression, a potentially hazardous diagnostic test in patients who are extremely ill or suffer from coronary artery disease.

Elective surgery should be postponed in all hyperthyroid subjects except those with very mild disease until the metabolic rate has been restored to normal with blocking drugs, radioiodine, or subtotal thyroidectomy. Propranolol, a beta sympathetic blocking drug that antagonizes the peripheral actions of thyroid hormone, is a useful agent for management of patients requiring emergency surgery.[13, 28, 47, 65] Tremulousness, excessive sweating, tachycardia, elevated pulse pressure, and other manifestations of hypermetabolism diminish. When administered in sufficient dosage, the drug is rapidly effective. Its action appears to be mediated solely via the adrenergic system, since iodine trapping by the gland and serum concentration of iodothyronines do not change.[13, 47] The dose of propranolol necessary for an adequate response varies with each patient,[65] ranging from 10 to 40 mg every 6 hours, and must be adjusted on an individual basis. Fatigue, weakness, depression and weight loss are generally not affected by this medication. Intravenous propranolol 2 to 5 mg every 10 to 30 minutes can be administered intraoperatively if necessary and should be continued in the postoperative period until the patient is able to take the medication by mouth.[65]

Beta sympathetic blocking drugs such as propranolol should be considered as adjunctive rather than primary medication in the preoperative and intraoperative management of thyrotoxic patients, unless there is insufficient time for the physician to prepare the patient with antithyroid medication. Of the medications effective in suppressing thyroid function, iodine is the most useful agent and acts rapidly via inhibiting release of thyroxine from the gland.[56, 59] One gram of sodium iodide can be added to a liter of intravenous solution and repeated every 12 hours. It should be noted that, under rare circumstances, in the presence of severe iodine deficiency, the administration of iodine may aggravate thyrotoxicosis by increasing intrathyroidal iodine concentration.[64] This agent should thus be used with caution and, whenever possible, in conjunction with other antithyroid drugs. If there is sufficient time, iodine should be administered for 7 to 10 days prior to surgery. Two drops of saturated solution of potassium iodide (SSKI) three times daily is sufficient to produce a maximum effect on inhibition of thyroxine secretion by the gland.[7] Adverse reactions to iodine are not unusual, but are generally not serious. These include an acneform skin rash, drug fever, sialoadenitis, conjunctivitis, and rhinitis. These reactions are reversible if the medication is discontinued.

The major agents employed in the chemotherapy of thyrotoxicosis are the thioamides propylthiouracil and methimazole.[32, 52] Although they also inhibit the coupling reaction, the principal mode of action of these agents is inhibition of oxidation and organic binding of thyroidal iodine. Both drugs have a relatively short half life (4 to 6 hours in plasma) and thus have to be administered every 6 to 8 hours.[44] When possible, these agents should be administered by mouth: 100 mg every 8 hours for propylthiouracil, 10 mg every 6 to 8 hours for methimazole. In patients with severe thyrotoxicosis or very large goiters, larger doses may have to be employed. The most serious side effect of these agents, bone marrow suppression, more commonly occurs with daily doses exceeding 300 mg for propylthiouracil and 40 mg for methimazole. Since these drugs inhibit synthesis rather than release of thyroxine by the thyroid gland, a clinical response occurs only after depletion of glandular hormone stores. This latent period can be reduced if larger doses of the drug are employed, although such a dosage schedule increases the risk of bone marrow suppression.

If there is sufficient time for optimal use of the thioamide drugs, the dose of either medication is adjusted to maximize effectiveness and minimize side effects. There is gradual amelioration of the symptoms and signs of thyrotoxicosis and reduction in the size of the goiter. The dose should be reduced after clinical response occurs, with the maintenance dose generally one half or less of the initial therapeutically effective dose. The appearance of hypothyroidism associated with an increase in the size of the goiter suggests excessive dosage of the drug.

Management of patients on thioamide drugs therefore requires clinical evaluation of the patient every 4 to 6 weeks and measurement of circulating T_4 and TSH levels every 2 to 3 months in order to avoid incipient hypothyroidism. In this author's experience, exophthalmus may be aggravated by excessive administration of thioamide medication and can be avoided by careful titration of the drug or concomitant administration of physiologic replacement doses of thyroxine.

Adverse reactions occur in a small percentage of patients taking thioamide medication. The most significant of these are skin rash, drug fever, joint effusions, and agranulocytosis. Fever and sore throat generally alert the physician to a significant decline in circulating leukocytes. These manifestations will clear with prompt interruption of medication. Agranulocytosis is the most serious of these drug reactions and occurs in approximately 0.3 percent of patients. Although more common during the first few months of treatment, this adverse reaction has been observed after several years of drug administration. Careful supervision of all patients on thioamides is therefore necessary, with complete blood counts measured at regular intervals and during any coexisting infection. Should agranulocytosis develop, the drug must be discontinued immediately and the patient isolated and treated with blood transfusions, corticosteroids, and appropriate antibiotics. Recovery almost always occurs, but generally takes 10 days to 2 weeks. Crossover reactions between propylthiouracil and methimazole occur with sufficient frequency to contraindicate a second trial of either thioamide if this serious drug reaction has developed.

Whenever time permits, propylthiouracil or methimazole and iodine should be administered for a sufficient period of time to render the patient euthyroid prior to surgery. If elective surgery can be postponed for several months, a subablative dose of radioactive iodine (4–6 mCi) or subtotal thyroidectomy offers the patient permanent cure of hyperthyroidism and avoids the risk attendant to prolonged administration of iodine and blocking drugs.[32, 41]

IATROGENIC HYPERTHYROIDISM

Iatrogenic hyperthyroidism develops in patients taking excessive quantities of thyroid hormone, either on the advice of a physician or surreptitiously. The diagnosis is suggested if typical clinical signs of hyperthyroidism and elevated plasma T_4 and T_3 concentration occur concomitant with a low uptake of radioiodine by the gland. Generally, hyperthyroidism in such patients is not sufficiently severe to compromise the patient's response to surgery, but alterations in requirements and metabolic clearance rates of anesthetic agents as a consequence of excess tissue concentrations of hormone need to be considered carefully by the anesthesiologist. In the presence of severe iatrogenic hyperthyroidism, surgery should be postponed if possible until the excess hormone has been metabolized. If emergency surgery is necessary, propranolol is the drug of choice to block the peripheral actions of excess thyroid hormone.

THYROTOXIC CRISIS

Thyrotoxic crisis (thyroid storm) is an extreme accentuation of both the signs and symptoms of thyrotoxicosis. This rare but extremely serious complication of thyrotoxicosis is associated with a high morbidity and mortality. The disorder has an abrupt onset, usually evoked by the stress of infection, trauma, or surgery in a patient with previously unrecognized and untreated hyperthyroidism. The clinical picture is dominated by the effects of excessive tissue concentration of thyroid hormone: sinus tachycardia or atrial fibrillation with rapid ventricular response, marked increase in systolic and pulse pressure, high temperature, profuse sweating, marked tachypnea, tremulousness, extreme restlessness, nausea, vomiting, and abdominal pain. Delirium and frank psychosis may occur. In a patient with heart disease, pulmonary edema and other signs of congestive heart failure develop. As the disorder progresses, apathy, stupor, and coma with hypotension supervene. If unrecognized and untreated, the condition is almost always fatal.

Treatment of thyroid storm aims to correct both the severe thyrotoxicosis and the underlying precipitating event. Treatment includes large doses of thioamide medication (200 mg of propylthiouracil or 20 mg of methimazole every 4 hours) orally or by stomach tube; iodine, administered as SSKI four drops every 4 hours orally, or sodium iodide, 1 to 2 g by slow intravenous infusion every 12 hours; and propranolol 40 to 400 mg every 3 to 6 hours orally or 2 to 5 mg intravenously every 30 to 120 minutes. Supportive measures include intravenous fluids, multivitamin and B vitamin complex, hydrocortisone 100 to 300 mg daily, antipyretic agents, cooling blanket or ice packs, and adequate sedation. Digitalis and diuretics are added if congestive heart failure is present. In the presence of thyrotoxic crisis or impending crisis, no surgical procedure can be safely performed. Treatment of thyroid storm generally requires 5 to 7 days before the manifestations of severe hyperthyroidism can be brought under control. If thyrotoxic crisis develops intraoperatively, propranolol should be administered in incremental doses intravenously with careful attention to supporting fluid balance, ventilation, oxygenation, and blood pressure; surgery should be interrupted as soon as feasible.

SUMMARY

Disorders of the thyroid gland are frequently unrecognized and untreated by the attending physician and present the anesthesiologist with a diagnostic and therapeutic challenge. Very large goiters distort and compress the larynx and require an experienced anesthesiologist for safe intubation. If surgery is elective and can be postponed in patients suspected of being hypo- or hyperthyroid, there is sufficient time to permit the anesthesiologist and the attending physician to obtain appropriate tests of thyroid function and institute appropriate therapeutic measures to restore the metabolic rate to normal. When there is insufficient time to confirm a clinical diagnosis of thyroid disease, the anesthesiologist is faced with important therapeutic decisions. It is the author's opinion that therapeutic intervention is, in most instances, preferable to therapeutic nihilism. In the case of a patient suspected of hypothyroidism, it is usually safe to administer a physiologic replacement dose of thyroxine to support the patient intraoperatively and postoperatively. If hypothyroidism is associated with cardiovascular disease, other debilitating illness, or advanced age, thyroxine must be given with extreme caution in order to avoid dangerous tachyarrhythmias or too rapid acceleration of the metabolic rate. The hyperthyroid patient facing nonelective surgery represents a very serious challenge to the anesthesiologist, since marked accentuation of clinical hyperthyroidism (thyroid storm) is a major risk of such surgery. In such a situation, intravenous propranolol and intravenous iodine are the optimal drugs for a safe and uncomplicated clinical course during and following surgery. In both instances, the anesthesiologist must use skillful clinical judgment in making the appropriate diagnosis and selecting appropriate therapy. Careful and continuous supervision of the patient is necessary during and following surgery and appropriate treatment and support of the patient should be provided until it is safe to discontinue therapy, if necessary, to confirm the diagnosis of thyroid disease. Careful clinical judgment and judicious use of appropriate medication should provide the patient with a smooth and safe intraoperative course and a rapid and uncomplicated postoperative recovery.

ACKNOWLEDGMENTS

The author wishes to acknowledge the assistance of Vivienne Grande, Research Assistant; Thomas Burk, Director, Medical Photography, Tucson Medical Center; and Thomas Moon, Ph.D., Chief, Biostatistics, University of Arizona Health Sciences Center, Cancer Center Division, in the preparation of this manuscript.

REFERENCES

1. Alexander, W. D., Koutras, D. A., et al.: *Quantitative studies of iodine metabolism in thyroid disease.* Q. J. Med. 31:281, 1962.
2. Anderson, M. D., Bowers, C. Y., et al.: *Synthetic thyrotropin releasing hormone. A potent stimulator of thyrotropin secretion in man.* N. Engl. J. Med. 285:1279, 1971.
3. Beckers, C., and Cornette, C.: *TSH production rate in non toxic goiter.* J. Clin. Endocrinol. 32:852, 1971.
4. Begg, T. B., and Hall, R.: *Iodine goiter and hypothyroidism.* Q. J. Med. 32:351, 1963.
5. Bellabarba, D., Inada, M., et al.: *Thyroxine transport and turnover in major non thyroidal illness.* J. Clin. Endocrinol. 28:1023, 1968.
6. Braverman, L. E., Ingbar, S. H., et al.: *Conversion of thyroxin (T_4) to triiodothyronine (T_3) in athyreotic human subjects.* J. Clin. Invest. 49:855, 1970.
7. Braverman, L. R., Vagenakis, A. G., et al.: *Studies on the pathogenesis of iodine myxedema.* Trans. Assoc. Am. Physicians. 84:130, 1971.
8. Buccino, R. A., Spann, J. F., et al.: *Influence of the thyroid state on the intrinsic contractile properties and energy stores of the myocardium.* J. Clin. Invest. 46:1669, 1967.
9. Challoner, D. R., and Allen, D. O.: *An in vitro effect of triiodothyro-*

nine on lipolysis, cyclic AMP-C14 accumulation and oxygen consumption in isolated fat cells. Metabolism, 19:480, 1970.

10. Chopra, I. J., Fisher, D. A., et al.: *Thyroxine and triiodothyronine in the human thyroid.* J. Clin. Endocrinol. 36:311, 1973.
11. Choufoer, J. C., Van Rhijn, M., et al.: *Endemic goiter in Western New Guinea. II. Clinical picture, incidence and pathogenesis of endemic cretinism.* J. Clin. Endocrinol. 25:385, 1965.
12. Cotton, G. E., Gorman, C. A., et al.: *Suppression of thyrotropin (h-TSH) in serums of patients with myxedema of varying etiology treated with thyroid hormone.* N. Engl. J. Med. 285:521, 1971.
13. Das. G., and Krieger, M.: *Treatment of thyrotoxic storm with intravenous administration of propranolol.* Ann. Intern. Med. 70:985, 1969.
14. DeGroot, L. J., Nagasaka, A., et al.: *Biosynthesis of thyroid hormone.* Excerpta Medica Int. Congr. Ser. 285:53, 1970.
15. DeLange, F., Hershmann, J. M., et al.: *Relationship between the serum thyrotropin level, the prevalence of goiter and the pattern of iodine metabolism in Idjwi Island.* J. Clin. Endocrinol. 33:261, 1971.
16. DeRubertis, F. R., Michelis, M. F., et al.: *Impaired water excretion in myxedema.* Am. J. Med. 51:41, 1971.
17. DiScala, V. A., and Kinney, M. J.: *Effects of myxedema on the renal diluting and concentrating mechanism.* Am. J. Med. 50:325, 1971.
18. Dumont, J. E.: *The action of thyrotropin on thyroid metabolism.* Vitam. Horm. 21:287, 1971.
19. Durie, B. G. M., Hellman, D. W., et al.: "Multimodality treatment of high risk thyroid carcinoma." From the Health Sciences Center, University of Arizona, Tucson, Arizona. In Salmon, S. E., and Jones, S. E. (eds.): *Adjuvant Therapy of Cancer.* Elsevier, North Holland Biomedical Press, Amsterdam, 1977.
20. Eayrs, J. T.: *Influence of the thyroid on the central nervous system.* Br. Med. Bull. 16:122, 1960.
21. Eayrs, J. T.: "Thyroid and central nervous system development." In *The Scientific Basis of Medicine Annual Reviews.* The Athlone Press, University of London, 1966, p. 317.
22. Edmonds, C. J., Hayes, S., et al.: *Measurement of serum TSH and thyroid in the management and treatment of thyroid carcinoma with radioiodine.* Br. J. Radiol. 50:799, 1977.
23. Emerson, D. H., Dyson, W. L., et al.: *Serum thyrotropin and thyroxin concentration in patients receiving lithium carbonate.* J. Clin. Endocrinol. 36:388, 1973.
24. Engel, A. H.: *Neuromuscular manifestations of Graves disease.* Mayo Clin. Proc. 47:9, 1972.
25. Friedman, M. J., Okada, R. D., Hellman, D., et al.: *Alterations in systolic and diastolic left ventricular function in man by serial com-*

puterized echocardiographic analysis during the hyperthyroid and euthyroid state. Western Society for Clinical Research, Carmel, California, February 7–9, 1979.

26. Gross, H. A., Appleman, M.D., et al.: *Effects of biologically active steroids on thyroid function in man.* J. Clin. Endocrinol. 33:242, 1971.
27. Grossman, W., Robin, N. I., et al.: *The enhanced myocardial contractility of thyrotoxicosis. Role of the beta adrenergic receptor.* Ann. Int. Med. 74:869, 1971a.
28. Grossman, W., Robin, N. I., et al.: *Effects of beta blockade on the peripheral manifestations of thyrotoxicosis.* Ann. Int. Med. 74:875, 197b.
29. Hellman, D.: Unpublished observations.
30. Hellman, D.: *Free thyroxine, total thyroxine and TSH: comparison in the diagnosis of clinical hypothyroidism.* In preparation.
31. Hermann, J. T., and Quarton, G. C.: *Psychological changes and psychogenesis in thyroid hormone disorders.* J. Clin. Endocrinol. 25:327, 1965.
32. Hershmann, J. M.: *The treatment of hyperthyroidism.* Ann. Int. Med. 64:1306, 1966.
33. Hilts, S. V., Hellman, D., et al.: *Serial TSH determination after T_3 withdrawal or thyroidectomy in the therapy of thyroid carcinoma.* J. Nucl. Med., September, 1979.
34. Hollander, C. S., Scott, R. L., et al.: *Increased protein-bound iodine and thyroxine-binding globulin in acute intermittent porphyria.* N. Engl. J. Med. 277:996, 1967.
35. Holvey, D. N., Goodner, C. J., et al.: *Treatment of myxedema coma with intravenous thyroxine.* Arch. Int. Med. 113:89, 1964.
36. Ingbar, S. H.: *Autoregulation of the thyroid. Response to iodine excess and depletion.* Mayo Clin. Proc. 47:814, 1972.
37. Lamki, L., Row, V. V., et al.: *Cell-mediated immunity in Graves disease and in Hashimoto's thyroiditis as shown by the demonstration of migration inhibition factor (MIF).* J. Clin. Endocrinol. 36:358, 1973.
38. Levey, G. S.: *Catecholamine sensitivity, thyroid hormone and the heart.* Am. J. Med. 50:413, 1971.
39. Mori, T., and Kriss, J. P. *Measurements by competitive binding radioassay of serum and anti-microsomal and anti-thyroglobulin antibodies in Graves disease and other thyroid disorders.* J. Clin. Endocrinol. 33:688, 1971.
40. Nicoloff, J. T., Lowe, J. C., et al.: *Simultaneous action of thyroxine and triiodothyronine peripheral turnover kinetics in man.* J. Clin. Invest. 51:473, 1972.
41. Nofal, M. M., and Beierwaltes, W. H.: *Treatment of hyperthyroidism with sodium iodide I^{131}.* J.A.M.A. 197:605, 1966.

42. Oddie, T. H., Fisher, D. A., et al.: *Iodine intake in the United States: a reassessment.* J. Clin. Endocrinol. 30:659, 1978a.
43. Oddie, T. H., Meade, J. H., Jr., et al.: *An analysis of published data on thyroxine turnover in human subjects.* J. Clin. Endocrinol. 26:425, 1966.
44. Pittman, J. A., Beschi, R. J., et al.: *Methimazole: its absorption and excretion in man and tissue distribution in rats.* J. Clin. Endocrinol. 33:182, 1971.
45. Ramsey, I.D.: *Muscle dysfunction in hypothyroidism.* Lancet, 2:931, 1966.
46. Reichlin, S., Martin, J. B., et al.: *The hypothalamus in pituitary-thyroid regulation.* Recent Prog. Horm. Res. 28:229, 1972.
47. Riddle, M. C., and Schwartz, T. G.: *New tactics for hyperthyroidism: a sympathetic blockade.* Ann. Int. Med. 72:749, 1970.
48. Royce, P. C.: *Severely impaired consciousness in myxedema—a review.* Am. J. Med. Sci. 261:46, 1971.
49. Ruder, H., Corvol, P., et al.: *Effects of induced hyperthyroidism on steroid metabolism in man.* J. Clin. Endocrinol. 33:382, 1971.
50. Sanders, V.: *Neurologic manifestations of myxedema.* N. Engl. J. Med. 266:547, 599, 1972.
51. Snyder, P. J., and Utiger, R. D.: *Response to thyrotropin releasing hormone (TRF) in normal man.* J. Clin. Endocrinol. 34:380, 1972a.
52. Solomon, D. H., Beck, J. C., et al.: *Prognosis of hyperthyroidism treated by antithyroid drugs.* J.A.M.A. 152:201, 1953.
53. Stanbury, J. B.: "Familial goiter." In Stanbury, J. B., Wyngaarden, J. B., et al. (eds.): *The Metabolic Basis of Inherited Disease.* McGraw-Hill, New York, 1972.
54. Strauss, H. W., Hurley, P. J., et al.: *Advantages of ^{99m}Tc pertechnetate for thyroid scanning in patients with decreased radioiodine uptake.* Radiology 97:307.
55. Torrigiani, G., Doniach, D., et al.: *Serum thyroglobulin levels in healthy subjects and in patients with thyroid disease.* J. Clin. Endocrinol. 29:305, 1969.
56. Vagenakis, A. G., Downs, P., et al.: *Control of thyroid hormone secretion in normal subjects receiving iodides.* J. Clin. Invest. 52:528, 1973.
57. Vannotti, A., and Beraud, T.: *Functional relationship between the liver, the thyroxine binding protein of serum in the thyroid.* J. Clin. Endocrinol. 19:466, 1959.
58. Wallack, M. S., Adelberg, H. M., et al.: *A thyroid suppression test using a single dose of l-thyroxine.* N. Engl. J. Med. 283:402, 1970.
59. Wartofsky, L., Ransil, B. J., et al.: *Inhibition by iodine of the release of thyroxine from the thyroid glands of patients with thyrotoxicosis.* J. Clin. Invest. 49:78, 1970.

60. Wilbur, J. F., and Utiger, R. D.: *The effect of glucocorticoids on thyrotropin secretion.* J. Clin. Invest. 48:2096, 1969.
61. Wilkins, L.: *Epiphyseal dysgenesis associated with hypothyroidism.* Am. J. Dis. Child. 61:13, 1941.
62. Wilson, W. R., and Bedell, G. N.: *The pulmonary abnormalities in myxedema.* J. Clin. Invest. 39:42, 1960.
63. Woeber, K. A., and Ingbar, S. H.: "The interaction of the thyroid hormones with binding proteins." In Gree, M. A., and Solomon, D. H. (eds.): *Thyroid, Handbook of Physiology.* American Physiologic Society, Washington, 1973.
64. Wolff, J.: *Iodide goiter and the pharmacologic effects of excess iodide.* Am. J. Med. 47:101, 1969.
65. Zonszein, J., Santangelo, R. P., Macklin, J. F., et al.: *Propranolol therapy in thyrotoxicosis. A review of 84 patients undergoing surgery.* Am. J. Med., 66:411, 1979.

10

ANESTHETIC IMPLICATIONS OF HYPERTHYROIDISM

Linda Stehling, M.D.

The classic "thyroid steal" is now an event of the past. In years past, at a time when there were no effective antithyroid or sympatholytic drugs, patients were surreptitiously given rectal tribromoethanol (Avertin) and "stolen" to the operating room under basal anesthesia conditions for thyroidectomy. Obviously times have changed. Thyroid storm can usually be prevented by adequate preoperative drug therapy. The introduction of beta adrenergic blocking drugs has changed the therapy and prognosis of the dreaded complication of thyroid storm if by chance it occurs in the unrecognized hyperthyroid patient scheduled for emergency surgery. Dr. Stehling's chapter complements Dr. Hellman's more basic chapter with a discussion of problems and solutions encountered with anesthetic management of patients with hyperthyroidism.

Burnell R. Brown, Jr.

MECHANISM OF ACTION OF THYROID HORMONES

Rational management of the thyrotoxic patient is based on a knowledge of the pathogenesis of the disease. Several mechanisms of thyroid hormone action have been put forth.[14, 15] They include:

1. Hormonally enhanced synthesis of proteins. Triiodothyronine has been shown to stimulate cellular protein synthesis in vivo and in cell cultures, but the effects on protein synthesis per se seem inadequate to account for the increased oxygen consumption characteristic of the disease.
2. Stimulation of the plasma membrane, enzyme Na^+-K^+-ATPase, the "sodium pump," is probably a major effect, but not the primary mechanism of thyroid hormone activity.
3. Activation of mitochondrial energy metabolism.
4. Enhanced activity of beta adrenergic stimuli at the level of the cell membrane. In favor of this theory are many of the clinical manifestations of thyrotoxicosis, which resemble excess adrenal medullary activity, amelioration of the symptoms by adrenergic blockade, and animal models suggesting an increased number of beta adrenergic receptor sites in cardiac plasma membranes.
5. Induced protein synthesis and turnover rates perhaps resulting from thyroid hormones acting as amino acid analogues.

It is likely that multiple mechanisms interact and that the effects on plasma membranes may be the initiating events, producing activation of mitochondrial energy metabolism and consequent increased oxygen consumption.

Many of the clinical manifestations of hyperthyroidism are related to compensatory mechanisms for dissipation of excess heat, e.g., profuse sweating, vasodilation, and tachycardia. A hyperkinetic circulatory state develops in which cardiac output is raised in excess of the requirements imposed by the hypermetabolic state. In addition to an accelerated heart rate, stroke volume is augmented and ventricular contractility is enhanced. These cardiovascular responses appear to be a direct effect of the thyroid hormones, perhaps independent of autonomic influences.

PHARMACOLOGIC MANAGEMENT

The majority of patients can be rendered euthyroid prior to operation. Exceptions include those who are hypersensitive to antithyroid drugs and patients in whom beta adrenergic blockade is contraindicated by asthma or a history of heart failure unrelated to thyroid disease. Rarely, airway obstruction will necessitate urgent thyroid surgery, but more commonly emergency surgery is performed for conditions unrelated to thyroid disease. A significant number of patients are unreliable and will not follow therapeutic regimens.

Thyrotoxicosis occurs in approximately 2 per 1000 pregnancies and therapeutic considerations involve mother and fetus.[1] Beta adrenergic blockade results in persistent stimulation of uterine musculature and has been reported to result in intrauterine growth retardation and a small placenta. However, its short-term use for preoperative preparation is presumably safe. Antithyroid drugs may also be used for preoperative preparation. If surgery is performed in the second trimester, the incidence of fetal wastage is not increased.[8]

In a very small percentage of patients, hyperthyroidism is the result of hormonal secretion by chorionic tissue of a hydatidiform mole or choriocarcinoma. Evacuation or removal of the uterus results in abrupt cessation of symptoms.

Antithyroid Drugs

When time and patient tolerance permit, the antithyroid drugs propylthiouracil or carbimazole may be administered. The mean time of onset of activity is 8 days, and 6 to 7 weeks are required before euthyroid status is achieved. In order to decrease the vascularity and hyperplasia of the gland and simplify surgical dissection, iodine is administered for 7 to 10 days prior to operation. However, patients who receive iodine therapy in excess of 2 weeks compensate to partially overcome the induced decrease in hormone secretion with gradual return toward pretreatment status, the phenomenon of "iodide escape." Thus, initiation of iodine therapy limits flexibility in the timing of surgery. Should surgery not be possible within 2 weeks, iodine is discontinued and at least 6 weeks are allowed to elapse prior to reinstitution of iodine therapy.

Beta Adrenergic Blockade

Propranolol (Inderal) is probably the most widely used agent for patients with thyrotoxicosis. The peripheral manifestations of the disease are usually dramatically improved within a few days of institution of therapy. The chronotropic and inotropic effects of excess hormonal secretion are greatly diminished and left ventricular efficiency is enhanced. Although the heart rate is slowed, it usually does not return to normal, suggesting that the circulatory changes of hyperthyroidism are mediated only in part through the beta sympathetic receptors and that thyroxine exerts independent activity on the myocardium.[10] It has been suggested that suppressed peripheral conversion of T_4 to T_3 may contribute to the effectiveness of propranolol; however, the inhibition is slower in onset than are the clinical effects. Cardiac output is reduced, but oxygen consumption remains unchanged. Drug requirements are highly variable; the conventional 160 mg/day given p.o. in four divided doses frequently does not provide adequate plasma levels.[3] Levels of 50 to 100 ng/ml are usually sufficient to confer beta blockade, but serial measurements of propranolol levels are not practical. In addition, levels are highly variable, especially in thyrotoxic patients.[11] Dosage should be adjusted to control the peripheral manifestations of the disease.

Discontinuation of the drug prior to surgery has been compared to omitting insulin in the diabetic. For some time after its introduction, anesthesiologists were wary of the myocardial depressant effects of propranolol. In a recent small series of patients treated preoperatively with the agent and anesthetized with halothane, Trench and associates[16] found a maximal decrease in cardiac output owing to decreased stroke volume of 21 percent, accompanied by a raised CVP and total peripheral resistance. A return to preoperative levels occurred by the end of surgery. The half-life of propranolol is 3.4 to 6 hours; therefore, discontinuing the drug 24 to 48 hours prior to operation allows sufficient time for recovery from blockade if desired.[2]

Advantages of treatment with propranolol include rapid symptomatic relief, a low failure rate, and flexibility in scheduling surgery, as iodine is not usually administered. Therapy must be continued 5 to 10 days following thyroidectomy. Current opinion is that the drug is a useful adjunct in the interim management of severe thyrotoxicosis. A conservative approach is expressed by Rubenfeld and associates,[11] who state that "until additional data relating propranolol levels to drug effects become available, caution should be used in treatment of thyrotoxic patients with propranolol alone."

Catecholamine Depletion

Prior to the advent of propranolol and in patients where the drug is contraindicated, use of the adrenergic blocking agents reserpine and guanethidine has proven effective. Definite clinical improvement occurs in most patients treated with reserpine. A decreased pulse rate is usually the first objective evidence of drug effect; blood pressure is little affected. The dose is .75 to 4 mg per day orally or 7.5 to 15 mg per day intramuscularly. Guanethidine has the advantage of not altering mental status, in contrast to the depressant effect of reserpine. It is preferred by some who associate changes in mental status with thyroid status. Heart rate, cardiac output, and cardiac work return toward normal, but oxygen consumption is not significantly lowered—another bit of evidence that the sympathetic nervous system is not responsible for the elevated oxygen consumption associated with thyrotoxicosis. The average daily dose of guanethidine is 80 mg.[13]

Corticosteroids

Corticosteroids may play a part in the preoperative preparation of patients. The mechanism of action is probably decreased peripheral conversion of T_4 to T_3, but may also be the result of suppression of TSH secretion or decreased secretion of thyroid hormones. Increased metabolic destruction of corticosteroids is associated with hyperthyroidism and a relative insufficiency may occur. There are case reports of patients rendered clinically euthyroid following administration of steroids alond.[13]

Timing of Surgery

Following 1 to 2 weeks of propranolol or 6 to 8 weeks of therapy with antithyroid drugs, the patient should be ready for surgery. Nervousness, tremor, and muscle weakness should no longer be present. Thyroid myopathy clinically evident as weakness of the proximal muscle groups and associated with abnormal electromyograms is frequent, although patients may not complain of symptoms unless queried specifically.

The resting pulse should be in the 80s or below at the time of surgery. The clinical status of the patient is more important than any absolute laboratory value. It is to be remembered that adrenergic blocking agents do not alter laboratory paramenters.

ANESTHETIC MANAGEMENT

Adequate premedication is essential. The agent of choice is diazepam administered orally. The best way to ascertain the proper dosage is by "trial premedication." The optimal dose can usually be arrived at by administering what is thought to be a dose that will induce moderate sedation and evaluating the patient 60 to 90 minutes later. If large doses do not produce the required degree of sedation, it is preferable to sedate the patient the night prior to surgery and to start a slow intravenous infusion. The intravenous route can then be used to administer additional medication in the patient's room prior to transfer to the operating room. The patient should be transported to the operating room in his own bed rather than being awakened and moved to a stretcher. Personnel must be made aware of the need for a smooth induction in a quiet room.

Anticholinergics are omitted because they interfere with the sweating mechanism. However, atropine has been utilized to confirm the adequacy of antithyroid therapy. It is alleged that patients may be considered euthyroid if 0.6 mg of atropine does not cause the pulse to increase by more than 30 beats per minute or exceed 120 beats per minute.[12]

Thiopental is the induction agent of choice. The thiobarbiturates possess antithyroid activity, presumably related to their thiocarbamate structure (N—C=S). In animals given a single large dose of thiopental (40 mg/kg), impairment of thyroid activity is virtually instantaneous and persists 6 to 7 days. Inhalation agents that stimulate the sympathoadrenal axis, such as diethyl ether and cyclopropane, are contraindicated. Hypercarbia must be avoided for the same reason. Although methoxyflurane has a depressant effect on the sympathoadrenal system, its potential nephrotoxicity limits its use. The author has employed halothane in numerous thyrotoxic patients; however, enflurane is preferable as it does not sensitize the myocardium to catecholamines. Should a balanced technique be employed, it is imperative that the patient be deeply anesthetized, so that surgical stimuli do not evoke an outpouring of catecholamines. In addition, it is difficult to differentiate the effects of light anesthesia from the effects of catecholamines released by the narcotics themselves. Whatever the technique, the patient must be adequately anesthetized prior to laryngoscopy and endotracheal intubation. Failure to ensure adequate anesthesia is associated with ventricular arrhythmias, most often PVCs.

Spinal anesthesia was used as a therapeutic modality for severe thyrotoxicosis in the 1940s. The spinal anesthesia was not administered to provide anesthesia for the surgical procedure. Rather, its purpose was blockade of the sympathetic innervation of the adrenal medulla, thereby reducing the secretion of epinephrine. Following establishment of a T_4 to T_5 sensory block, general anesthesia was induced.[6]

Monitoring

In addition to monitoring heart tones and respiration with a precordial and/or esophageal stethoscope, observation of the ECG and frequent measurement of the blood pressure are mandatory. Continuous temperature monitoring by the rectal, esophageal, or tympanic route is essential. It is to be remembered that most patients become cold in the cool ambient temperature of the operating room and even a modest elevation in temperature (0.5–1°C) should be regarded with suspicion.

A cooling blanket, refrigerated intravenous solutions, and ice should be readily available. Corticosteroids, propranolol, chlorpromazine, and nitroprusside should be easily accessible.

COMPLICATIONS

Thyroid Storm

Monitoring must not cease with termination of the surgery. Thyroid storm, when related to surgery, usually develops within 6 to 18 hours postoperatively. It is characterized by hyperpyrexia, tachycardia, and susceptibility to severe hypotension. Prior to the advent of antithyroid drugs and adrenergic blocking agents, "storm" was rather frequent and was associated with a high mortality rate. It has been stated that thyroid storm is not a complication of the disease, but rather an intrinsic feature of hyperthyroidism in its most severe form. Therapy includes parenteral administration of sodium iodide, corticosteroids, and adrenergic blocking agents. Propranolol should be titrated carefully in doses of 0.5 to 1 mg intravenously. Supportive therapy includes provision of a high inspired oxygen concentration, aggressive cooling, adequate fluid replacement, ample caloric intake, and close observation, preferably in an intensive care unit. Improvement usually beings within a few hours of institution of therapy.

The thyrotoxic patient undergoing emergency surgery requires expert management if thyroid storm is to be averted. Recognition of the endocrinopathy may be difficult, as acute pathology or trauma may mask hyperthyroidism. The patient may be unaware of the problem or incapable of transmitting information. Propranolol is used to bring the pulse rate into the near-normal range. Rarely, hypertension occurs and nitroprusside can be used to lower peripheral resistance. Sodium iodide (0.5–3 g/day) and corticosteroids (hydrocortisone hemisuccinate (1–3 g/day) are administered intravenously.

Carotid Sinus Reflex

Severe hypotension with marked bradycardia or asystole may occur as a result of manipulation of the carotid sinus. Treatment consists of cessation of the stimulus and infiltration of the area around the bifurcation of the common carotid artery with a local anesthetic. Intravenous administration of atropine may also be beneficial.

Venous Air Embolism

Although uncommon, venous air embolism may occur if a large vein is opened. It has been stated that as much as 200 ml of air can be aspirated during a deep inspiration.[7]

Nerve Injury

A most feared complication, injury to the recurrent laryngeal nerves, may be bilateral or unilateral. The latter is usually tolerated, but damage to both nerves may necessitate tracheostomy. Injury of the superior laryngeal nerve results in loss of sensation in the larynx and piriform sinus. Aspiration is often associated with loss of sensory innervation.

Hypocalcemia

It is widely believed that hypocalcemia following thyroidectomy is the result of parathyroid damage. Prospective studies of thyrotoxic patients have demonstrated evidence of bone disease in the majority of patients. Negative calcium balance is due in part to large losses via stool and urine. Thyroid hormones also exert a primary effect on bone, decreasing calcium absorption and increasing its turnover. The net result of these factors is removal of calcium from bone.[9] It is proposed that acute reversal of the osteodystrophy immediately following thyroidectomy results in avid retention of calcium by bone and the signs of hypocalcemia. The role of thyrocalcitonin release remains to be established, since temporary falls in serum calcium have also been associated with thyroid surgery for disorders other than thyrotoxicosis.[19] Therapy is rarely required.

Permanent hypoparathyroidism is uncommon if surgical dissection is meticulous. Transient hypocalcemia as a result of damage to the vascular supply of the parathyroids is usually manifest within 24 to 72 hours. The intrinsic muscles of the larynx are exquisitely sensitive to calcium deficiency and inspiratory stridor may be the first manifestation of hypoparathyroidism, occurring long before overt tetany. Therapy consists of intravenous calcium chloride or calcium gluconate.

Miscellaneous Complications

Hematoma, tracheal malacia following removal of a large gland, laryngeal edema, laceration of the trachea, tracheoesophageal fistula, pneumomediastinum, pneumothorax, and phrenic or cervical sympathetic nerve injury can occur in association with thyroidectomy. If there is any question of damage to the recurrent laryngeal nerves, laryngoscopy should be performed at the termination of the procedure. In order to prevent laryngospasm or bucking on the tube, the preferred method is to extubate the spontaneously breathing but deeply anesthetized patients's trachea. In order to offer an additional margin of safety, it is best to extubate the trachea 3 to 5 minutes following discontinuation of nitrous oxide. The pharynx is suctioned, enflurane and oxygen continued, the laryngoscope inserted, and the endotracheal tube withdrawn. Only then is the anesthetic discontinued. Once vocal cord movement (or its absence!) is ascertained, the laryngoscope is withdrawn and the patient's ventilation assisted by mask if necessary.

CONCLUSION

In this era of malignant hyperpyrexia, hyperthyroidism is rarely discussed and tachycardia and an elevated temperature may be misdiagnosed. Hyperthyroid patients whose disease is recognized can usually be rendered euthyroid prior to operation. Some patients are unaware of the diagnosis, others refuse to follow therapeutic regimens, and yet others require emergency surgery for nonrelated conditions. A high index of suspicion, careful monitoring, and selective pharmacologic manipulation are required for optimal management of the hyperthyroid patient.

REFERENCES

1. Burrow, G. N.: *Maternal-fetal considerations in hyperthyroidism.* Clin. Endocrinol. Metab. 7:115–125, 1978.
2. Faulkner, S. L., Hopkins, J. T., Boerth, R. C., et al.: *Time required for complete recovery from chronic propranolol therapy.* N. Eng. J. Med. 289:607–609, 1973.
3. Hellman, R., Kelly, K. L., and Mason, W. D.: *Propranolol for thyroid storm.* N. Eng. J. Med. 297:671–672, 1977.
4. Howitt, G., and Rowlands, D. J.: *Beta-sympathetic blockade in hyperthyroidism.* Lancet 1:628–631, 1966.
5. Howitt, G., Rowlands, D. J., Leung, D. Y., et al.: *Myocardial contractility and the effects of beta-adrenergic blockade in hypothyroidism and hyperthyroidism.* Clin. Sci. 34:485–495, 1968.
6. Knight, R. T.: *The use of spinal anesthesia to control sympathetic overactivity in hyperthyroidism.* Anesthesiology 6:225–230, 1945.
7. Kritchman, M. M., and Papper, E. M.: "Anesthesia in thyroid disease." In Werner, S. C., and Ingbar, S. H. (eds.): *The Thyroid.* ed.3. Harper & Row, New York, 1971, pp. 481–488.
8. Levy, C. A., Waite, J. H., and Dickey, R.: *Thyrotoxicosis and preg-*

nancy: use of preoperative propranolol for thyroidectomy. Am. J. Surg. 133:319–321, 1977.

9. Michie, W., Duncan, T., Hamer-Hodges, D. W., et al.: *Mechanism of hypocalcaemia after thyroidectomy for thyrotoxicosis.* Lancet 508–513, March 1971.
10. Pietras, R. J., Real, M. A., Poticha, G. S., et al.: *Cardiovascular response in hyperthyroidism.* Arch. Intern Med. 129:426–429, 1972.
11. Rubenfeld, S., Silverman, V. E., Welch, K. M. A., et al.: *Variable plasma propranolol levels in thyrotoxicosis.* N. Engl. J. Med. 300:353–354, 1979.
12. Shires, G. T.: *Questions and answers on anesthesia for thyroid surgery.* Clin. Anesth. 1:206, 1963.
13. Stehling, L. C.: *Anesthetic management of the patient with hyperthyroidism.* Anesthesiology 41:585–595, 1974.
14. Sterling, K.: *Thyroid hormone action at the cell level. Part 1.* N. Engl. J. Med. 300:117–123, 1979.
15. Sterling, K.: *Thyroid hormone action at the cell level. Part 2.* N. Engl. J. Med., 300:173–177, 1979.
16. Trench, A. J., Buckley, F. P., Drummond, G. B., et al.: *Propranolol in thyrotoxicosis. Cardiovascular changes during thyroidectomy in patients pre-treated with propranolol.* Anaesthesia 33:535-539, 1978.
17. Verhoeven, R. P., Visser, T. J., Docter, R., et al.: *Plasma thyroxine, 3,3′,5-triiodothyronine and 3,3′,5′-triiodothyronine during B-adrenergic blockade in hyperthyroidism.* J. Clin. Endocrinol. Metab. 44:1002–1005, 1977.
18. Wase, A. W., and Foster, W. C.: *Thiopental and thyroid metabolism.* Proc. Soc. Exp. Biol. Med. 91:89–91, 1956.
19. Wilkin, T. J., Paterson, C. R., Isles, T. E., et al.: *Post-thyroidectomy hypocalcaemia: a feature of the operation or the thyroid disorder?* Lancet 621–623, March 1977.

SURGERY OF THE PARATHYROID GLANDS

Hugo V. Villar, M.D., and
Stephen L. Wangensteen, M.D.

The authors of this chapter, both surgeons, have had considerable experience managing parathyroid endocrinopathies. As they note, parathyroid surgery and anesthesia may constitute the most common category of endocrine operative procedure performed. A good overview of pre- and postoperative management is described. While the authors do not allude to specific anesthetic drugs, their review succinctly describes the pathophysiologic consequences of abnormalities of the parathyroid glands in such a way that logical conclusions regarding anesthetic requirements can be reached.

Burnell R. Brown, Jr.

Disorders of the parathyroid glands, both hyper- and hypoparathyroidism, present a special problem for the anesthesiologist and the surgeon. In the first place, hyperparathyroidism can be difficult to diagnose. In addition, the dangers of hypercalcemia, dehydration, mental confusion, renal colic, bone disease, gastrointestinal bleeding, and pancreatitis may tremendously complicate the management of the patient. On the other hand, the diagnosis of hypoparathyroidism is relatively simple. The patient is usually aware of the problem and the physician can easily identify it. The symptoms are usually dramatic and are related to tetany with laryngeal spasm, anxiety, and possible renal colic.

Hyperparathyroidism has slowly emerged as a relatively common disease. In order to fully understand this disease it is imperative to have knowledge of the metabolism of calcium and phosphorus in the body.[11, 18]

The body contains about 1000 g calcium, which is stable in bone; 11 g is in the cells; 1 g is in the extracellular fluid. The average daily intake of calcium is about 0.5 to 1 g; the daily average urinary calcium excretion is about 300 to 400 mg. Calcium absorption takes place principally in the duodenum and upper jejunum and is an active process involving vitamin D. In plasma, about 40 percent of the calcium is ionized. Another 40 percent is protein bound, and the remainder is complexed to organic anions as citrate and phosphate. The level of ionized calcium is most relevant because it determines most metabolic functions. Calcium levels play a critical role in determining the excitability of nerve function and the contractability of skeletal and cardiac muscle. It is also important in the structure and function of cell membranes and organelles and in numerous cellular metabolic events, including hormone release. Rasmussen believed there was a close relationship between calcium anion and the action of cyclic adenosine monophosphate (cAMP).[18] Since it is difficult to measure ionized calcium concentration for clinical purposes, total serum calcium concentrations are used. They usually correlate quite well as long as serum protein concentrations are normal. In an abnormal state, for each gram of alteration of total protein above or below 6.5 g/100 ml, there is a 1 mg/100 ml increase or decrease in protein-bound calcium. Normal serum calcium concentrations range from 9 to 10.5 mg/100 in most laboratories. The kidneys normally reabsorb 90 percent of the filtered calcium. The maximum capacity of the kidney to excrete calcium is about 500 mg per day. Therefore, if marked hypercalcemia is present, either from bone destruction, from metastasis, or from increased secretion of parathyroid hormone, the kidney may be unable to increase calcium excretion, and serum calcium will rise. If renal damage is present, this function is even more compromised and serum calcium will rise to even greater levels.

The adult body contains about 700 g of phosphate, most of which is located in the bones and teeth. Plasma phosphate measures 2.5 to 4.3 g/100 ml. The plasma levels of calcium and phosphate vary inversely one with the other and normally the relationship is such that the product of plasma calcium and phosphate is constant and ranges between 30 and 40. In contrast to calcium, serum phosphate values change markedly with diet and age (higher in children). Phosphate absorption takes place in the midintestine. Absorption is increased by parathyroid hormone (PTH), growth hormone, vitamin D, and a low calcium diet. It is decreased by aluminum hydroxide ingestion. Most of the phosphate is excreted in the urine.

MAGNESIUM METABOLISM

The body contains about 200 mEq magnesium, mostly in the skeleton. Absorption is increased by vitamin D and renal excretion and levels closely follow those of calcium. Hypomagnesemia occurs in hyperparathyroidism, alcoholism, malnutrition, and prolonged intravenous hyperalimentation if magnesium is not added to the feeding regimen. Severe hypomagnesemia frequently occurs after resection of a parathyroid adenoma, even when the plasma levels have been normal preoperatively. Normal magnesium levels are about 1.5 to 2.5 mg/100 ml. Mental confusion and even tetany may be caused by hypomagnesemia. Some cases of refractory tetany cannot be corrected until serum magnesium levels are returned to normal.

Two polypeptides, parathyroid hormone (molecular weight 9500) and calcitonin (molecular weight 3600), are the principal hormones regulating calcium metabolism. Secretion of PTH is inversely related to plasma calcium concentration. The main effects of PTH are on bone and kidney. In the skeleton it causes a shift of calcium from bone to the extracellular fluid, thereby raising serum calcium levels. In the kidney, PTH increases tubular excretion of phosphate and enhances calcium reabsorption; thus the main effects of PTH are hypercalcemia and hyperphosphaturia. The homone activity is mediated by cyclic 3′,5′ adenosine monophosphate (3′,5′ AMP), produced through specific hormonal activation of the enzyme adenyl cyclase in bone and kidney. [3]

The primary action of calcitonin is to inhibit bone reabsorption, thereby lowering the serum calcium concentration. It is produced by the C cells (parafollicular cells) of the thyroid gland. These cells are part of the APUD system of peptides or amine-secreting cells described by Pearse and Polak.[16] Radioimmunoassay of calcitonin is important in the diagnosis of occult medullary carcinoma of the thyroid in man.

VITAMIN D

The natural form of vitamin D is called vitamin D_3 or cholecalciferal. It is produced by irradiation of 7-dihydrocholesterol in the skin. To be metabolically active, D_3 should first be hydroxylated in the liver and further in the kidney. [14] It has been suggested that vitamin D acts as a physiologic hormone that has a feedback control mechanism. In the presence of parathyroid hormone, when serum calcium or serum phosphorus levels are low, there is an increased synthesis of active vitamin D, which then makes calcium and phosphorus available from the bone and intestine. Vitamin D increases the reabsorption of calcium from the intestine.

HYPERPARATHYROIDISM

Hyperfunction of the parathyroid gland is now established as one of the most common endocrine disorders seen by the anesthesiologist and the surgeon. Unfortunately, the diagnosis remains a problem on occasion. The cause of spontaneous hyperfunction of the parathyroid gland is unknown. As with many endocrine neoplasms, overactivity is recognized not because of an anatomic enlargement, but because of the peripheral effects of excess hormone. Primary hyperparathyroidism most commonly develops between 35 and 65 years of age. It is three times more common in females, especially in postmenopausal women. The most common cause (85%) is a chief cell adenoma.

Water clear cell adenomas are much less frequent. The incidence of primary chief cell hyperplasia is debated. Its incidence varies from 5 to 20 percent, depending on the pathologic interpretation. The discrepancies are due to different operative approaches, different pathologic interpretation, and the incidence of patients with familial hyperparathyroidism, multiple endocrine adenomatoses, and chronic kidney dialysis in each series. Carcinoma of the parathyroid is quite rare and accounts for about 1.5 percent of the causes of primary hyperparathyroidism. In about 90 percent of the cases the disease is functional and will be revealed by marked elevated serum calcium. The radioimmunoassay for parathyroid hormone has proved very useful in the differential diagnosis of hypercalcemic states. Normal plasma levels are about 200 pg/ml. PTH levels should always be interpreted in conjunction with serum calcium levels.

The common use of automatic analyzers for chemical entities in blood plasma has posed a special problem regarding the diagnosis of hypercalcemia. On routine analysis many patients are found to have elevated calcium levels and depressed phosphorus, while being asymptomatic. If several calcium levels are below 11 mg, a conservative approach is warranted. On the other hand, if the serum calcium levels are greater than 13 mg, despite the absence of symptoms or complications, it is advisable to go ahead with the neck exploration.[4, 10, 13, 15, 17, 20, 25]

Signs and Symptoms of Hyperparathyroidism

Hypercalcemia with hypercalcinuria and hypophosphatemia and hyperphosphaturia are common findings. Three main groups of symptoms are found: hypercalcemic, renal, and gastrointestinal. Hypercalcemia is responsible for muscle weakness and extreme fatigue. As the calcium level rises, muscular relaxation increases. Patients may be unable to hold things with their hands. With calcium levels above 16 mg percent, even cardiac standstill may occur. Mental confusion and coma may occur with levels around 16 to 17 mg/100. This confusion may be mistaken for cerebral vascular accident. Nausea, anorexia, constipation, polyuria, and polydipsia are all secondary to hypercalcemia. A hypercoagulation state mainly caused by severe dehydration has also been reported in some patients.

Renal complications are generally the most severe clinical

manifestations of hyperparathyroidism. About 65 percent of patients will have nephrolithiasis. [24] Patients usually complain of back pain, hematuria, and the passing of renal calculi. Most of the calculi are composed of calcium phosphate or calcium oxalate. Nephrocalcinosis is much less common, occuring in about 10 percent of patients. It is uncommon for nephrocalcinosis and nephrolithiasis to occur together. Renal damage is much more common in patients with evidence of nephrolithiasis and nephrocalcinosis, but it may occur even in the absence of renal calcification. This renal damage is usually irreversible, even after the hyperparathyroidism has been corrected. About 80 to 90 percent of patients with hyperparathyroidism have some impairment of renal function.

Musculoskeletal symptoms usually are mild and vague and include weakness, hypertonia, and joint pain, but in severe cases of bone involvement, actual fractures or shortening of stature may occur. Subperiostial reabsorption in the phalange of the hand (Fig. 1) is common. Bone cysts and osteoclastomas are also a distinct finding, usually in the medullary part of the shaft of long bones, metacarpals, and ribs.

In patients with multiple endocrine adenomatosis a higher incidence of peptic ulcer disease has been reported, as well as a more virulent course of their ulcer diathesis. [12] Bleeding and perforation have been reported in patients with severe hypercalcemia. In hypercalcemic patients with severe peptic ulcer disease, therapy should be aimed first at correction of the hypercalcemia, by removal of the hyperparathyroid adenoma, rather than the performance of gastric surgery. The incidence of pancreatitis in patients with hyperparathyroidism also seems increased.

Proper preoperative management of patients with hypercalcemia is crucial.[9, 21] Careful attention to rehydration is a cardinal step in the preoperative preparation. Liberal use of physiologic electrolyte solutions and glucose is mandatory. Preoperative BUN, creatinine, and specific gravity of the urine are mandatory in order to evaluate the degree of dehydration and renal function. A marked discrepancy between BUN and creatinine will generally be a good index of prerenal dehydration and, therefore, of the need for vigorous fluid therapy. On the other hand, a low specific gravity in the urine could be misleading and only be an indication of renal damage and inability of the kidney to

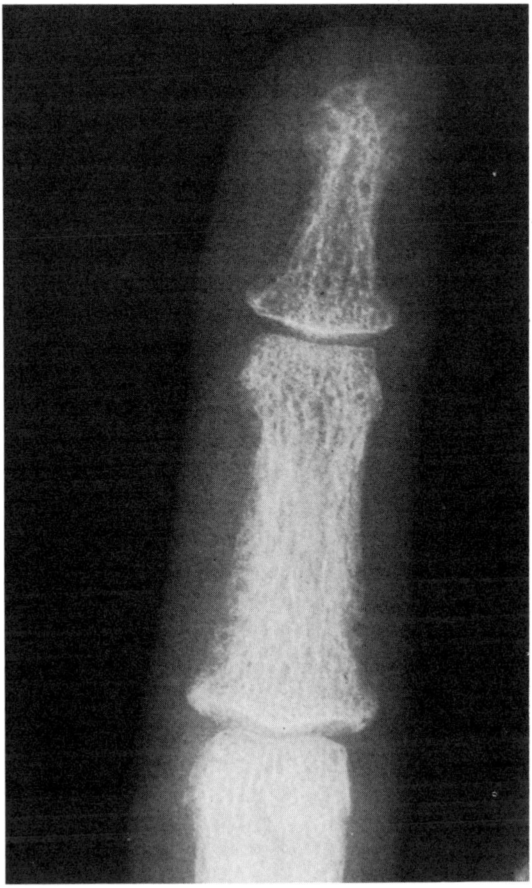

Figure 1. Subperiosteal reabsorption of the cortices of the middle phalanges is pathognomic for hyperparathyroidism. Note the loss of distal phalangeal tuft cortex, loss of demarcation between cortex and medulla, and general deossification. (Courtesy of Dr. Michael G. Pitt, Department of Radiology, AHSC.)

concentrate. Rehydration of the patient should be started at least 24 to 36 hours before the planned surgery. Hypokalemia is frequently present and may require replacement of large amounts of potassium for correction.

Calcium and digitalis are synergistic in effect on the myocardium and conducting system; therefore, it may be necessary to reduce or stop digitalis. Similarly, if digitalization is required on hypercalcemic patients, a lower dose is generally required.

Since, in most instances, calcium excretion parallels sodium excretion, natriuresis will enhance calcium excretion. [22] The combination of large amounts of isotonic saline solution plus furosemide gives excellent results. Fluid electrolytes and cardiovascular status should be carefully monitored to avoid overloading and severe hypokalemia.

DIFFERENTIAL DIAGNOSIS OF HYPERCALCEMIA

It has long been known that on occasion neoplasms may produce a variety of polypeptides, such as ACTH, melanocyte-stimulating hormone (MSH), follicle-stimulating hormone (FSH), antidiuretic hormone (ADH), and insulin. It is now clear that some tumors also produce a PTH-like circulating hormone and/or prostaglandins, each of which may result in hypercalcemia. [1] The most common causes of hypercalcemia are

- Bone Metastases
- Primary Hyperthyroidism
- Ectopic Hyperthyroidism
- Miscellaneous
  - Thiazides
  - Vitamin D Intoxication
  - Sarcoidosis
  - Milk-Alkali Syndrome
  - Thyrotoxicosis

Malignancy with bone metastasis accounts for over 50 percent. This is usually due to the secretion of PTH-like substance by the malignant tumor. Squamous cell carcinoma of the lung, oat cell carcinoma of the lung, hypernephromas, and carcinoma of the ovaries are the most common malignancies associated with hypercalcemia.

SECONDARY HYPERPARATHYROIDISM

A frequent complication of patients with chronic renal failure who have been maintained on dialysis or have undergone renal transplantation has been the development of secondary hyperparathyroidism. [7] Serum calcium levels are not elevated; metastatic calcifications and a variety of bone lesions are usually present. Medical management is quite unsatisfactory and removal of the hyperplastic parathyroid gland is usually required.

Preoperative and postoperative examinations of the vocal cords should be performed in all patients undergoing parathyroid and major thyroid surgery. Generally, preoperative indirect laryngoscopy is done, and usually the anesthesiologist can observe the movement of the vocal cords upon removal of the endotracheal tube.

ANESTHESIC CONSIDERATIONS IN HYPERCALCEMIC PATIENTS

No single anesthetic technique is superior in parathyroid surgery. Preparation should be made for a prolonged, tedious exploration of the neck because of the need for indentification of all four parathyroid glands. On occasion even the mediastinum may be opened. A blood-free operative field is facilitated by use of the head-up position of the patient, keeping in mind that this position increases the possibility of air embolism.

From clinical experience, circulatory complications do not seem to be frequent or severe during removal of hyperfunctioning glands, even in those patients with severe hypercalcemia. Theoretically, excessive serum calcium might be expected to have adverse effects on the heart; however, Bronsky and associates [2] found no change in cardiac rate or rhythm in 35 patients with hypercalcemia. The electrocardiogram may show a prolonged PR interval at levels greater than 16 mg. T waves become prolonged and rounded and the QT interval becomes quite long (Fig. 2). Increased susceptibility to digitalis is present in hypercalcemic patients.

The possibility of an accidental pneumothorax during the neck exploration should be kept in mind.

No neuromuscular changes have been reported. Significant effects of muscle relaxant drugs in the presence of hypercalcemia have not been found. However, since high calcium ions are known to affect membrane transport, potentiation of muscle relaxants could be expected in theory.

POSTOPERATIVE MANAGEMENT

The postoperative management of a patient after parathyroid surgery can be complicated. The need for rehydration is still present in the first 48 to 72 hours. If airway problems are found in the immediate postoperative period, a hematoma in the neck

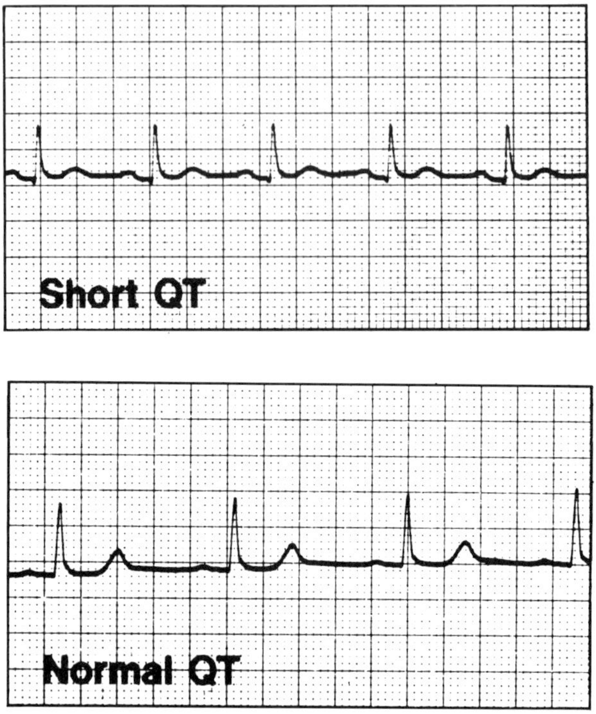

Figure 2. Electrocardiogram of a 55-year-old woman with metastatic carcinoma of the breast. Serum calcium was 17.5 mg/100 ml. Notice short QT interval. (Courtesy of Dr. Gordon A. Ewy, Department of Internal Medicine, AHSC.)

compressing the trachea must be investigated. Close collaboration with the surgeon in the accurate diagnosis of the airway problem is mandatory.

The low calcium diet mandatory prior to the operation should be continued postoperatively for the first 2 to 3 days. The rate and the level at which the calcium falls gives a clue regarding the adequacy of the resection of the parathyroid tissue. The magnitude of the fall is an indication of the future need for calcium and of the skeletal deficit. Serum calcium reaches its lowest level in about 48 to 72 hours after parathyroid surgery and returns to normal 2 to 3 days thereafter. The sooner after surgery the drop in serum calcium occurs and the longer it persists, the greater the likelihood that all parathyroid glands have been damaged, and the poorer the prognosis for recovery of function. A second contributing factor in the drop of serum calcium after parathyroid surgery is the degree of bone decalcification. If there has been significant decalcification during the active phase of the disease, the skeleton will require calcium repletion after the operation. If calcium is not available in the diet in an adequate amount, the calcium levels in the blood may fall to levels producing tetany. This is the most common cause of severe tetany encountered after surgery for hyperparathyroidism. Elevated preoperative alkaline phosphatase levels are an indicator of the severity of bone disease. Correction of the hyperparathyroidism alters the adverse balance between destruction and construction. Bone recalcification proceeds rapidly, reaching a peak 3 weeks after surgery. Addition of calcium and vitamin D will facilitate the rebuilding process. Calcium may be given as lactate 300 to 900 mg four times daily and vitamin D is given 50,000 to 100,000 units per day. If medication cannot be given orally, calcium gluconate may be given intramuscularly or intravenously.[5, 6, 8, 19, 23]

The major signs and symptoms of hypocalcemia are directly attributable to the reduction of plasma ionized calcium, which leads to an increased neuromuscular excitability. Clinically, the earliest manifestations are numbness and tingling in the perioral area, fingers, and toes. Mental symptoms are common and patients are anxious, depressed, and occasionally confused. If tetany develops, carpopedal spasms, tonic convulsions, and laryngeal spasms may occur. Laryngeal spasms may be fatal.

Patients should not be discharged until an adequate evaluation of the calcium deficit is made and an adequate oral replacement is started.

Bone cysts, brown tumors, osteoporosis, fractures, and bone pain usually diminish quickly after removal of a parathyroid adenoma.

Sometimes in the postoperative period a stone or two lodged in the renal pelvis may break up, become dislodged, and impinge upon the ureter. Patients should be warned of the possibility of a kidney stone in the immediate postoperative period.

A few patients may experience an acute attack of gout, usually in the toes but sometimes in the ankles and wrists. In many patients the uric acid level rises slightly in the first days after operation and is most likely responsible for the development of gout. This pseudogout also disappears promptly and requires no specific treatment.

SUMMARY

Surgical procedures involving the parathyroid glands pose special problems. Careful attention to preoperative rehydration, control of hypercalcemia, and evaluation of renal function are mandatory. Intraoperative management is usually uncomplicated. Severe hypocalcemia may complicate the postoperative period, especially if severe bone disease is present.

REFERENCES

1. Ackerman, N. B., and Winer, N.: *The differentiation of primary hyperparathyroidism from the hypercalcemia of malignancy.* Ann. Surg. 181:226, 1975.
2. Bronsky, D., Dubin, A., Waldestein, S. S., et al: *Calcium and the electrocardiogram. Electrocardiographic manifestations of hyperparathyroidism and of marked hypercalcemia from various other etiologies.* Am. J. Cardiol. 7:833, 1961.
3. Cohn, D. V., MacGregor, R. R., Chu, L. L., et al.: *Biosynthesis of proparathyroid hormone and parathyroid hormone: chemistry, physiology and role of calcium in regulation.* Am. J. Med. 56:767, 1974.
4. Cope, O.: "The parathyroid glands." In Kinney, J. M., Egdahl, R. H., and Zuidema, G. D. (eds): *Manual of Preoperative and Postoperative care.* ed.2. W. B. Saunders Co., Philadelphia, 1971, pp. 482–504.
5. Edis, A. J.: *Surgical anatomy and technique of neck exploration for primary hyperparathyroidism.* Surg. Clin. North Am. 57:495, 1977.
6. Edis, A. J., Beahrs, O. H., van Heerden, A. J., et al.: *"Conservative" versus "liberal" approach to parathyroid neck exploration.* Surgery 82:466, 1977.
7. Glassford, M. D., Remmers, A. R., Sarles, H. E., et al.: *Hyperparathyroidism in the maintenance dialysis patient.* Surg. Gynecol. Obstet. 142:329, 1976.
8. Goldsmith, R. S.: *Physiology for physicians: hyperparathyroidism.* N. Engl. J. Med. 281:367, 1969.
9. Goldsmith, R. S.: *Treatment of severe hypercalcemia.* Med. Clin. North Am. 56:951, 1972.
10. Hines, J. R., and Suker, J. R.: *Unusual manifestations of parathyroid disease.* Surg. Clin. North Am. 53:221, 1978.
11. Kaplan, E. L.: "Recent advances in calcium metabolism: application

to medullary carcinoma of the thyroid and hyperparathyroidism." In Nyhus, L. M. (ed.): *Surgery Annual.* Appleton-Century-Crofts, New York, 1973, pp. 97-119.
12. Linos, D. A., van Heerden, J. A., Abboud, C. F., et al.: *Primary hyperparathyroidism and peptic ulcer disease.* Arch. Surg. 113:384, 1978.
13. Mallette, L. E., Bilezikian, J. P., Heath, D. A., et al.: *Primary hyperparathyroidism: clinical and biochemical features.* Medicine 53:127, 1974.
14. Norman, A. W.: *1,25-Dihydroxyvitamin D_3: a kidney-produced steroid hormone essential to calcium homeostasis.* Am. J. Med. 57:21, 1974.
15. Paloyan, E., Paloyan, D., and Pickleman, J. R.: *Hyperparathyroidism today.* Surg. Clin. North Am. 53:211, 1973.
16. Pearse, A. G. E., and Polak, T. M.: *Cytochemical evidence for the neural crest origin of mammalian ultimobranchial C cells.* Histochemie 27:96, 1971.
17. Purnell, D. C., Scholz, D. A., and Smith, L. H.: *Diagnosis of primary hyperparathyroidism.* Surg. Clin. North Am. 57:543, 1977.
18. Rasmussen, H.: *Ionic and hormonal control of calcium homeostasis.* Am. J. Med. 50:567, 1971.
19. Satava, R. M., Beahrs, O. H., and Scholz, D. A.: *Success rate of cervical exploration for hyperparathyroidism.* Arch. Surg. 110:625, 1975.
20. Schwartz, I. I., and Kaplan, E. L.: "Thyroid and parathyroid." In Schwartz, S. I. (ed.): *Principles of Surgery.* ed.3. McGraw Book Co. New York, 1979.
21. Schweitzer, V. G., Thompson, N. W., Harness, J. K., et al.: *Management of severe hypercalcemia caused by primary hyperparathyroidism.* Arch. Surg. 113:373, 1978.
22. Suki, W. N., Yium, T. T., Von Minder, M., et al.: *Acute treatment of hypercalcemia with furosemide.* N. Engl. J. Med. 283:836, 1970.
23. Wang, C. A.: *Parathyroid re-exploration.* Am. J. Surg. 186:140, 1977.
24. Williams, H. E.: *Physiology in medicine: nephrolithiasis.* N. Engl. J. Med. 290:33, 1974.
25. Wells, S. A., Jr.: "The parathyroid glands." In Sabiston, D. C. (ed.): *Textbook of Surgery.* ed. 11. W. B. Saunders Co., Philadelphia, 1977, pp. 725–738.

12

INFLUENCE OF GENERAL ANESTHESIA AND SURGICAL STRESS ON ENDOCRINE FUNCTION

T. Oyama, M.D.

Professor Oyama has been very active in investigating the phenomenology of endocrine responses during various types of anesthesia and surgery. It is interesting that anesthetic drugs and adjuvants do not alter endocrine responses greatly. The major factor in altering endocrine responses seems to be surgery, not our anesthetics. The following article surveys the changes reported.

Burnell R. Brown, Jr.

Endocrine and metabolic responses to anesthesia and surgical stress play an important role in the intra- and postoperative course of the patient. These responses are greatly modified by the condition of the patient preoperatively, including the general or specific nutritional state of the patient, presence or absence of injury, fluid and electrolyte balance, magnitude of surgical stress, and type of anesthetic management.

In this chapter consideration will be given to some endocrine changes during and following planned and controlled operations under general anesthesia. It is emphasized that the influence of anesthesia on endocrine function is actually less than the influence of the surgery itself. It should also be remembered that endocrine disease exerts an influence on the course of anesthesia and surgery.

A thorough understanding of the endocrine and metabolic responses of patients during anesthesia and the postoperative period is beneficial to rational anesthetic management. The subjects to be covered are (1) the hypothalamic-hypophyseal-adrenal cortical axis (ACTH, cortisol, aldosterone, renin); (2) growth hormone, insulin, glucagon; (3) thyroid hormone; and (4) sex hormone.

THE HYPOTHALAMUS AND PITUITARY

There are many hypothalamic nuclei that produce and secrete releasing factors (RF), which in turn stimulate the pituitary to produce or release corresponding trophic hormones. Releasing factors pass into the portal hypothalamohypophyseal circulation and are thus able to exert their effects rapidly on the anterior lobe of the pituitary while in relatively high concentration. The pituitary trophic hormones stimulate peripheral endocrine organs and influence the activity of the corresponding hypothalamic nuclei by either a negative or positive feedback mechanism, and so regulate pituitary function (Fig. 1).

Postoperative metabolic changes are demonstrable in the form of negative nitrogen balance, sodium retention and potassium loss, reduced glucose tolerance, and increased plasma concentration of free fatty acids. It is possible that the general endocrine response to stress is a nonspecific reaction. The role of hormones in the metabolic responses to the surgical

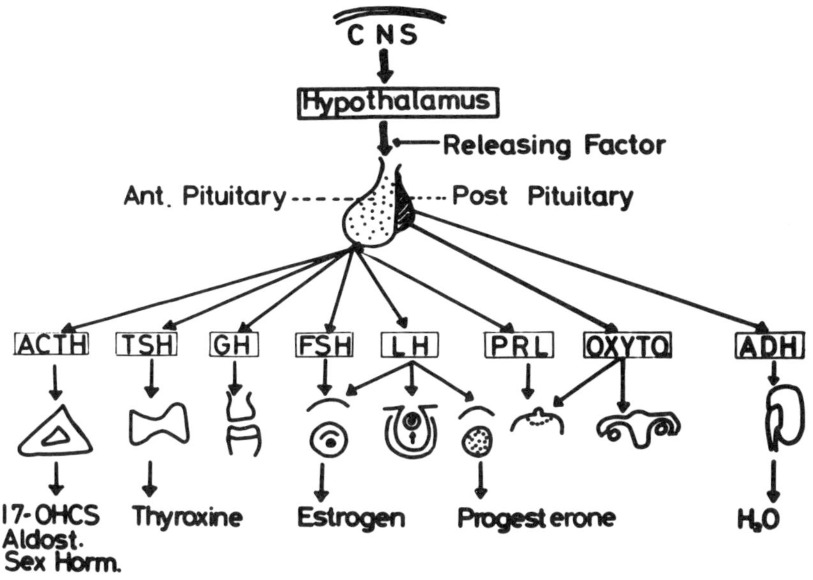

Figure 1. Schematic illustration of the role of the pituitary in stimulation of endocrine glands.

trauma appears to be not negligible. The precise significance of the pronounced increase in cortisol production observed during stress has not yet been understood. It is also unknown whether there is an increased requirement for the hormones involved in the endocrine response to stress.

ADRENOCORTICOTROPHIN (ACTH)

ACTH in human plasma is increased markedly during induction of anesthesia and throughout surgery. Large amounts of ACTH are released intermittently.[5] In contrast, the level of cortisol in the plasma increases gradually. These effects are observed during administration of diethyl ether, halothane, gamma-hydroxybutyrate, and neuroleptanesthesia (droperidol and pentazocine) in man. No appreciable rise in plasma ACTH level has been detected during surgery carried out with spinal anesthesia, but the level increased markedly when the spinal anesthetic ended.

CORTISOL

The term cortisol will be used to mean unconjugated steroid, both protein-bound and unbound (free). Bound steroids appear to be physiologically inactive and act as a reservoir for the free forms. The concentration of plasma cortisol at any moment is determined primarily by its secretion, distribution, utilization, and degradation. It is generally agreed that the response of plasma cortisol to surgical trauma is mainly due to stimulation of the pituitary-adrenal system resulting in an increased secretion from the adrenal gland.

Preoperative emotional reactions, fear and apprehension, cause adrenocortical stimulation.[3] It has also been reported that sleeplessness enhances adrenocortical activity in man. Sedatives used for preanesthetic medication reduce the adrenocortical stimulation caused by preoperative emotional stress in the operating room just before induction of anesthesia. Furthermore, the sedative effectiveness of preanesthetic medication correlates well with the decrease in plasma cortisol levels. Effective agents include pentobarbital (2.0 mg/kg), hydroxyzine (2.5 mg/kg), diazepam (0.2 mg/kg), and nitrazepam (0.2 mg/kg), but meperidine (2.0 mg/kg i.m. 1 hour prior to anesthesia) does not inhibit adrenocortical stimulation caused by preoperative emotional stress.

Diethyl ether is the strongest stimulant to adrenocortical activity of the various anesthetic agents. It appears that neither a deep plane of anesthesia nor a duration of over 1 hour is necessary to produce significant adrenocortical stimulation by ether. Surgical stress evokes a marked rise of cortisol during anesthesia with ether as with almost all other anesthetics. Anesthesia with cyclopropane and halothane was found to be associated with a marked elevation of plasma cortisol in man (Fig. 2).

Methoxyflurane anesthesia alone for 30 minutes does not increase plasma cortisol levels, and enflurane slightly decreases them. Thiopental combined with nitrous oxide and muscle relaxant either decreases or has no influence on plasma cortisol levels. Propanidid alone (5.0 mg/kg for induction) has no influence, but ketamine (2.0 mg/kg for induction) combined with nitrous oxide does significantly stimulate adrenocortical activity.

Meperidine (50–250 mg for induction) combined with nitrous

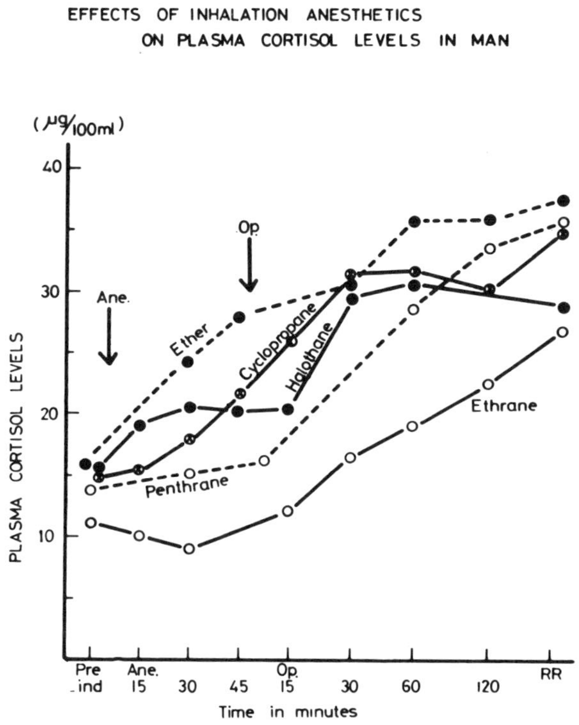

Figure 2. Plasma cortisol levels during anesthesia and surgery in man. "Op." denotes time surgery started.

oxide and neuroleptanesthesia, consisting of droperidol (0.15 mg/kg) and nitrous oxide followed with meperidine (20 mg), does not significantly influence adrenocortical function. Droperidol (0.15 mg/kg) plus pentazocine (1.0 mg/kg), supplemented with nitrous oxide, raises plasma cortisol. Droperidol (0.15 mg/kg) plus fentanyl (0.003 mg/kg for induction), followed by nitrous oxide and oxygen with fentanyl (0.05 mg intravenously as needed), does not increase plasma cortisol during anesthesia. Thus it would seem that the opiate antagonist pentazocine is responsible for the adrenocortical stimulation. Massive doses of morphine have been shown to inhibit increases in plasma cortisol concentration during surgery. The steroid anesthetic agent, Althesin (0.125 ml/kg), does not appreciably change plasma cortisol levels in man, and the normal adrenocortical response to surgical operations is observed.

Insofar as the muscle relaxants are concerned, the steroid-base pancuronium bromide has no significant effect on adrenocortical function in man. This is true of *d*-tubocurarine and succinylcholine also.

ALDOSTERONE AND PLASMA RENIN ACTIVITY

Plasma aldosterone concentrations (Fig. 3) in plasma are only about 1/2000th that of cortisol. Plasma concentrations of aldosterone in man are elevated 2.5 times greater than control values during ether-nitrous oxide anesthesia, 1.5 times during halothane-nitrous oxide, 1.6 times during methoyxflurane-nitrous oxide anesthesia, and 2 times during enflurane-nitrous oxide anesthesia, compared with control values (Fig. 3). There were

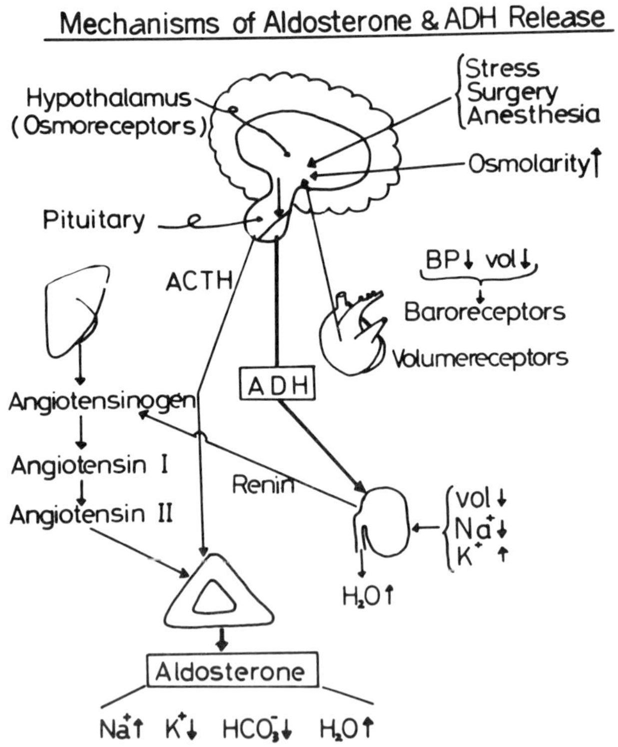

Figure 3. Relationships of pituitary, ADH, and renin-angiotensin systems.

further increases (about 3 times greater than control) at 0.5 to 2 hours after the start of surgery. Continuously elevated plasma concentrations of aldosterone were observed on the first pre-operative day. They returned to preanesthetic control values by the seventh postoperative day. A significant decrease in urinary Na/K ratio was associated with the increase in plasma aldosterone levels. Renin activity in the plasma was elevated slightly during ether-nitrous oxide and halothane-nitrous oxide anesthesia and surgery; however, no significant changes were observed in serum sodium or potassium concentrations.

Aldosterone is an important hormone, which influences fluid and electrolyte homeostasis. It causes increased tubular reabsorption of sodium and excretion of potassium, which decreases urinary excretion of sodium and chloride and increases that of potassium and thus expands the extracellular fluid compartment. Plasma levels of aldosterone are influenced by many factors. Influences include secretion from the zona glomerulosa of the adrenal cortex, metabolism in the liver, peripheral utilization, and renal excretion. However, adrenal secretion appears to play the main role in regulating plasma aldosterone concentration during stress. Aldosterone secretion is increased by ACTH, depletion of sodium, increase of potassium, a fall in the plasma sodium-to-potassium ratio, and reduction in the extracellular fluid or blood volume (Fig. 4).

A reduction of either blood volume or blood pressure, or vasoconstriction of the renal arteries, decreases the afferent arteriole pressure, which leads to a release of renin from the juxtaglomerular cells of the kidney. The renin converts angiotensinogen manufactured in the liver to angiotensin I.

This substance is further converted in the blood stream by an enzyme to angiotensin II, which stimulates the adrenal cortex to release aldosterone. Therefore, plasma renin activity is proportional to plasma concentration of angiotensin.

Aldosterone causes sodium retention and a rise in blood pressure. This acts as a feedback mechanism to shut off the further release of renin. It is not, however, certain whether this feedback mechanism operates during stress. In our study the plasma renin activity did not increase during anesthesia, but it rose significantly with surgery. According to Naruse,[1] plasma renin activity (PRA) was not changed during the early part of the operation. PRA did not change during halothane anesthesia.

Therefore, the participation of the renin-angiotensin system in elevated plasma aldosterone levels during anesthesia appears to be minor. However, it may play a role in elevated plasma aldosterone levels during surgery (Fig. 4).

Secretion of aldosterone is enhanced by falling plasma sodium and rising potassium levels. However, it seems unlikely that changes in plasma electrolyte levels are a major regulatory mechanism during anesthesia and surgery, since it appears that the changes must be relatively large before any stimulating effect is seen. In the dog the plasma potassium level must rise by at least 1 mEq/L or the plasma sodium fall by about 20 mEq/L before rises in aldosterone can be measured.

INSULIN, GROWTH HORMONE, AND GLUCAGON

Carbohydrate homeostasis is intimately associated with endocrine activity, particularly that of insulin and glucagon, which are secreted from the β and α cells of the pancreas. Other hormones such as cortisol, catecholamines, and pituitary growth hormone are also involved in carbohydrate homeostasis.

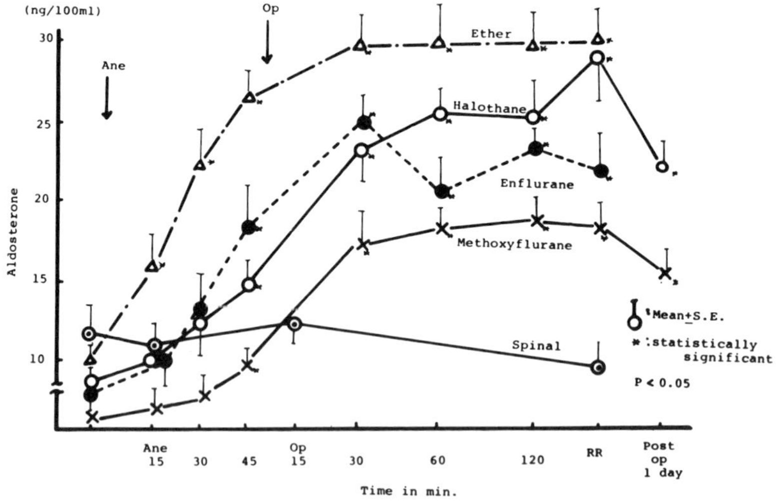

Figure 4. Plasma aldosterone levels during anesthesia and surgery in man. "Op" denotes time surgery started.

Insulin is important in promoting glucose uptake in fat and muscle cells. It also promotes the action of glycogen synthetase in the liver and enhances glycogen formation. Catecholamines and glucagon stimulate conversion of the phosphorylase enzyme system and accelerate glycogenolysis. Growth hormone, catecholamines, and glucagon stimulate conversion of the phosphorylase enzyme system and accelerate glycogenolysis. Growth hormone, catecholamines, glucocorticoids, and glucagon promote lipolysis and free fatty acid mobilization. Utilization of amino acids either as fuel in tricarboxylic acid cycle or in the liver to form glucose is promoted by catecholamines, glucocorticoids, and particularly by glucagon. Therefore, glucagon is important in regulating gluconeogenesis from amino acids.

Growth hormone (GH) increases protein synthesis and spares protein breakdown through gluconeogenesis. It reduces peripheral utilization and uptake of glucose, impairs glucose tolerance, increases retention of glucogen, decreases glucolysis, and has antiinsulin properties. The net actions of GH induce hyperglycemia.

Ether anesthesia in man is associated with an increase in plasma glucose levels. The mechanisms responsible for this effect probably include hepatic glycogenolysis, decreased tissue glucose utilization, and decreased renal glucose clearance. Plasma growth hormone concentrations fell during anesthesia and surgery, but rose significantly in the postoperative period.[4]

Halothane and enflurane anesthesia cause hyperglycemia, although the effects of these anesthetics are less marked than that of ether. Plasma GH levels during anesthesia alone increased slightly and rose significantly during surgery.

Anesthesia alone for 45 minutes with neuroleptanesthesia (droperidol and pethidine or pentazocine) and methoxyflurane increases plasma growth hormone levels from preinduction levels of 1.4 to 1.8 mμg/ml to 6 to 14 mμg/ml. Cyclopropane, thiopental, enflurane, and spinal anesthesia, however, do not increase growth hormone concentrations. The reasons for this difference in response to the various anesthetic agents are unknown.

Plasma glucagon levels decrease insiginificantly (24%) following pure halothane anesthesia for 30 minutes. They increase to 1.3 times control at 30 minutes after the start of surgery, with the peak level of 1.6 times over control found in the recovery room. Neuroleptanesthesia (droperidol, fentanyl, and nitrous oxide for 30 minutes) increased the plasma glucagon level to 1.3 times control, and further elevation was found 30 minutes after the start of surgery (1.6 times). The peak level (1.7 times control) was detected in the recovery room. A similar pattern of increased blood glucose in both groups was found during anesthesia and surgery. The precise mechanism of the different responses of plasma glucagon to both anesthetics is not known.

THYROID STIMULATING HORMONE (TSH) AND THYROXINE

Pituitary TSH levels in human plasma do not change appreciably during ether, halothane, methoxyflurane, thiopental, or spinal anesthesia. Thyroid hormones mainly consist of throxine (T_4) and triiodothyronine (T_3). Plasma concentration of T_3 is 1 to 2 percent that of T_4, but T_3 and T_4 exert almost the same activity because the biologic potency of T_3 is five times that of T_4. No significant variations in plasma TSH levels have been noted during anesthesia and surgery. Ether (25%) and halothane (12%), however, increase serum thyroxine levels, while methoxyflurane causes no change. Thiopental and spinal anesthesia decrease serum thyroxine concentrations. With ether or halothane anesthesia, surgery is usually associated with a rise in serum thyroxine. However, decreased serum thyroxine levels were found during surgery with thiopental or spinal anesthesia, although the magnitude of the surgical stress in these cases was less than that with the inhalation anesthetics.

All inhalation anesthetics including ether, halothane, methoxyflurane, and enflurane decreased (10–15%) plasma T_3 level in man. It was reduced further during surgery, and it decreased to 50 percent of the control level on the first postoperative day. Even on the seventh postoperative day, 30 percent reduction in plasma T_3 level was noted. Intravenous anesthetics, including thiopental and various types of neuroleptanesthetics combined with morphine, diazepam-ketamine, or diazepam-pentazocine, reduced plasma T_3, as did the inhalation anesthetics.

TESTOSTERONE

Testosterone not only affects sex function, but also influences metabolism as an anabolic hormone. Testosterone concentration in man falls 12 to 15 percent with various anesthetic agents, including halothane, thiopental-nitrous oxide, droperidol, and pentazocine.[2] It falls further during surgery to approximately 80 percent of preinduction levels. The lowest value (about 50%) is detected on the first postoperative day. Low concentrations of plasma testosterone persist for 1 week postoperatively.

The mechanism by which the peripheral venous testosterone concentration is reduced by anesthesia and surgery is unclear. However, the effect is probably directly on testicular function, rather than on an indirect pathway through the pituitary. The plasma concentration of luteinizing hormone (LH) is usually increased during anesthesia and surgery. LH is decreased in the postoperative period for at least 1 week, and the lowest levels occur on the seventh postoperative day (70% of the preinduction control level). The decreased testosterone secretion for 1 week might contribute to the well-known postoperative catabolic tendency.

Pituitary LH and FSH in adult females stimulate growth of the ovarial follicle, ovulation, and the formation of corpus luteum. These hormones stimulate ovarian secretion of estradiol and luteal progesterone, which regulate normal sexual function and the menstrual cycle. The author and colleagues studied the effect of halothane-N_2O anesthesia and hysterectomy on plasma LH, FSH, and estradiol levels in 30 female patients with regular menstrual cycles. The average age was 42 ± 1 (S.E.). The changes in plasma concentrations of these hormones during anesthesia and surgery suggest that in female surgical patients in midfollicular or midluteal phases, the variation of plasma levels of sex hormones appears to show a similar pattern as the normal menstrual phases. In contrast with male patients, the increase in plasma LH levels during surgery and the decrease in the postoperative period was not detected in female patients. Plasma concentration of testosterone in normal females is almost 1/20th that of the male. The maximal decrease recorded was 25 percent of control value on the third postoperative day.

REFERENCES

1. Naruse, T.: *Clinical studies on the variation of plasma aldosterone during surgery.* J. Jpn. Soc. Surg. 72:608, 1970.
2. Oyama, T., Aoki, N., and Kudo, T.: *Effect of halothane anaesthesia*

and surgery on plasma testosterone levels in men. Anesth. Analg. 51:130, 1972.
3. Oyama, T., Kimura, K., Takazawa, T., et al.: *An objective evaluation of tranquilizers as preanaesthetic medication: effect on adrenocortical function.* Can. Anaesth. Soc. J. 16:209, 1969.
4. Oyama, T. and Takiguchi, M.: *Effects of neuroleptanaesthesia on plasma levels of growth hormone and insulin.* Br. J. Anaesth. 42:1105, 1970.
5. Oyama, T. Takiguchi, M., and Kudo, T.: *Metabolic effects of anaesthesia: effect of thiopental-nitrous oxide anaesthesia on human growth hormone and insulin levels in plasma.* Can. Anaesth. Soc. J. 18:442, 1971.

13

ANESTHESIA FOR PHEOCHROMOCYTOMA

Burnell R. Brown, Jr., M.D., Ph.D.

The perioperative management of patients with pheochromocytoma constitutes one of the more challenging pharmacologic and physiologic exercises for the anesthesiologist. Although there is still some aura of mystique about diagnosis and therapy of this functioning adrenal medulla tumor, sound handling is predicated upon nothing more than a solid appreciation of the pathophysiologic consequences of altered adrenergic pharmacology. To illustrate this point with substantive data, it must be stated that in the 1940s, mortality rate of patients operated for pheochromocytoma approached 50 percent. Recent statistics indicate that the death rate is now less than 3 percent. It is the author's contention that this decline in mortality is due to both a better appreciation of the effects of long-term elevated catecholamines on the cardiovascular system and increased knowledge of the sympathetic nervous system and drugs that alter it.

BIOSYNTHESIS AND METABOLISM OF CATECHOLAMINES IN PHEOCHROMOCYTOMA

Pheochromocytomas are tumors of chromaffin tissue. Although a few of these tumors are nonfunctional, the vast majority secrete excessive amounts of catecholamines into the systemic circulation. Knowledge of the synthesis of catecholamines is essential to understanding the role and diagnostic implications of the various catecholamines produced by these tumors. Figure 1 illustrates the synthesis pathway. Tyrosine, the precursor, is converted to dihydroxyphenylalanine (dopa) by the enzyme tyrosine hydroxylase. This is the rate-limiting step of the entire reaction. Norepinephrine is defined as the sympathetic transmitter, stored in granules in postganglionic adrenergic nerves. Tumors of adrenergic nerves can be pure norepinephrine secretors. The enzyme phenylethanolamine-N-methyltransferase, which methylates norepinephrine to epinephrine, is in the adrenal tissue. Adrenal gland tumors can liberate both norepinephrine and epinephrine because of the presence of this enzyme.

Dopamine is the precursor of both epinephrine and norepinephrine. Mature pheochromocytomas do not ordinarily secrete a great deal of dopamine; however, malignant degenerate tumors can release large quantities of it. Therefore, urinary excretion of large amounts of dopamine and its metabolite, homova-

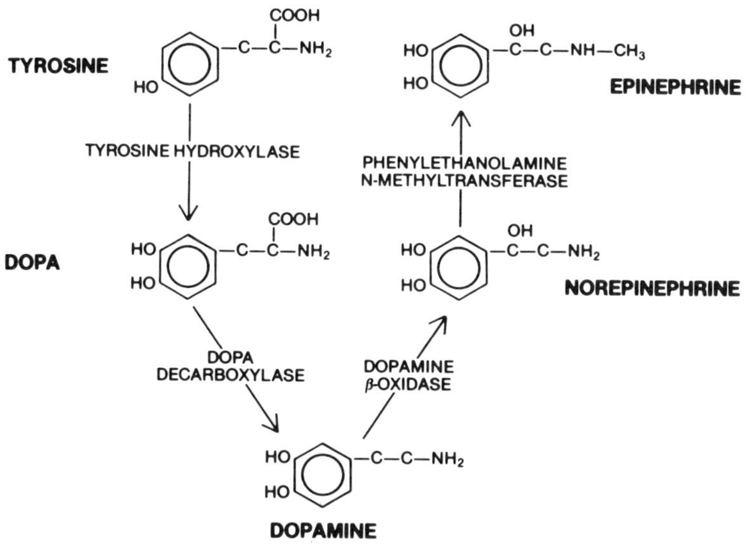

Figure 1. Biosynthesis of catecholamines.

nillic acid, in the urine can be a clue that malignant pheochromocytoma is present.

It is now well recognized that termination of action of catecholamines is achieved by means of a biophysical process, that is, active uptake into adrenergic nerve terminals. Clinically, if a single injection of epinephrine or norepinephrine is administered intravenously, pharmacologic activity and plasma levels decline within a few minutes owing to the rapid uptake of the amines into the sympathetic nerves. Metabolism of catecholamines does occur, but it is a rather slow process that is not proximally responsible for pharmacologic deactivation. However, the urinary metabolites of catecholamines give valuable insight into size and activity of pheochromocytomas.

Two enzymes participate in the biodegradation of catecholamines. Catechol-O-methyl transferase (COMT) is an enzyme found in high concentrations in plasma and liver. It converts both norepinephrine and epinephrine into O-methyl derivatives that are inactive (Fig. 2). Monoamine oxidase (MAO) is an intracellular enzyme, ordinarily associated with mitochondrial membranes. It functions to deaminate catecholamines, also inacti-

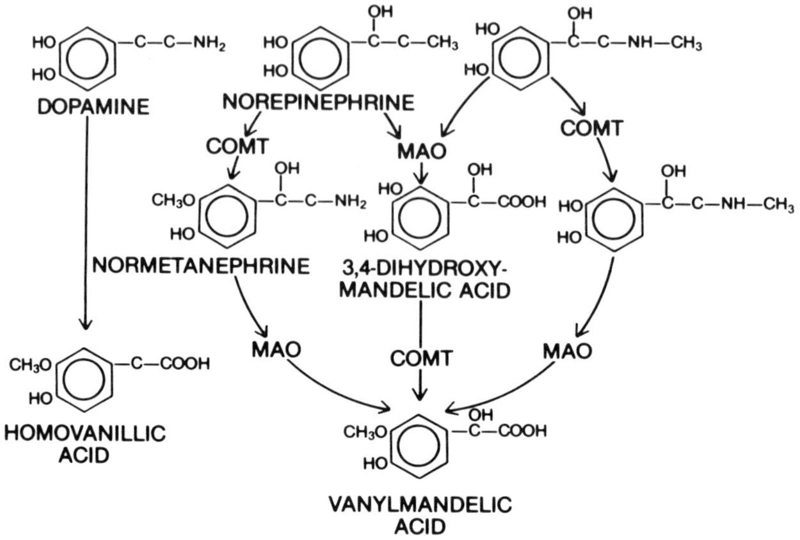

Figure 2. Scheme of enzymatic metabolism of catecholamines.

vating them. Customarily both enzymes attack a molecule of catecholamine sequentially. The final common product, the deaminated and O-methylated derivative, is vanylmandelic acid (VMA). Diagnosis of pheochromocytoma is heavily dependent on urinary catecholamines and metabolic products.[6] Patients are placed on a VMA-free diet (e.g., no bananas or vanilla) and urine is collected for 24 hours in hydrochloric acid. Both metabolites and free catecholamines are then quantitated. Normal 24-hour urinary excretion values of catecholamines and metabolites are shown in Table I. As will be described later in detail, urinary catecholamines and metabolites can be employed to determine tumor character, size, and location.[8]

Table 1. Normal 24-Hour Urinary Excretion of Catecholamines and Catecholamine Metabolites.

Norepinephrine	10–70 μg
Epinephrine	0–20 μg
Metanephrine	<1.3 mg
VMA	1.8–9.0 mg

PATHOPHYSIOLOGY OF PHEOCHROMOCYTOMA

Pheochromocytoma is an underdiagnosed condition: autopsy experience indicates it may be as common as 1 per 2000 of all autopsies.[4] Many symptoms of the tumor are rather protean and mimic essential hypertension or psychologic pathology. Sudden release of catecholamines from the tumors produces tachycardia, hypertension, dizziness, sweating, and anxiety. Effects of long-term elevated catecholamine concentrations include abnormal psychologic states, constipation, and sustained hypertension. Any patient with hypertension and abnormal behavior should be suspected of being a victim of this functioning tumor. Since catecholamines enhance glycogenolysis, the patient with pheochromocytoma may present as a mild diabetic. Fasting blood sugar levels of 130 to 160 mg/dl are not uncommon. Consistently elevated catecholamines may result in myocardiopathy, which will manifest as congestive heart failure.

One of the more insidious and dangerous problems seen with pheochromocytoma is reduction of red blood cell and plasma volume.[1] In other words, sustained levels of catecholamines over a period of time can produce a state of hypovolemia. Since the vasoactive catecholamines raise blood pressure, this hypovolemic state is masked. Initially, catecholamines constrict restrictive and capacitance vessels. This, in turn, causes a reduction in plasma volume. Red blood cell production is then decreased. Eventually, there is a decrease in total circulating volume. If the tumor is excised, the short half-life of the catecholamines will cause an immediate decrease in the vasoconstriction, and hypovolemia will become manifest as shock. Years ago, ignorance of this phenomenon was responsible for the high mortality rate associated with excision of pheochromocytomas. Instead of treating the rapid drop in blood pressure associated with removal of the tumor volume, it was felt the vascular system, "used to high catecholamines levels," necessitated more vasopressor. Use of a sympathomimetic amine in this situation did produce a better reading on the sphygmomanometer, but also caused decreased tissue perfusion and eventually severe acidosis and death. The unrecognized, preexisting hypovolemia undoubtedly accounted for many of the deaths. Although a decrease in circulating volume is not always associated with pheochromocytoma, it is quite common and represents a severe threat to body homeostasis if not recognized and corrected. Perhaps all patients scheduled for pheochromocytoma removal should be suspected of hypovolemia preoperatively. A clue that hypovolemia may exist is a high hematocrit (>46%), which indicates a deficiency of plasma volume.

CLASSIFICATION OF PHEOCHROMOCYTOMA

Although there may be considerable overlap, two rather distinct types of patients with pheochromocytoma are seen. These two groups can be distinguished by age, associated diseases, and tumor size.

SMALL TUMORS

These are defined as tumors with weights of approximately 30 g. Small pheochromocytomas are generally seen in younger patients (< 35 years of age). There is frequently a strong family history of pheochromocytoma, hypertension, and other endocrinopathies (Sipple's syndrome). These associated endocrinopathies include parathyroid adenoma and thyroid cancer. Functioning parathyroid adenoma should be searched for in most patients with pheochromocytoma by assessment of calcium metabolism. Parathyroid adenomas are not as life threatening as pheochromocytoma, so removal of them should be delayed for 4 to 6 weeks after surgery for the catecholamine-secreting tumor. All pheochromocytomas store catecholamines, which can be released into the systemic circulation spontaneously or by surgical manipulation. Small tumors usually store less catecholamines than large ones, but there are less enzymes present in the former. This fact dictates that, as a percentage, more "free" catecholamines than catecholamine metabolites are released by small tumors. If the ratio of urinary catecholamine metabolites/free catecholamines is compared, small tumors have a lower ratio (17 ± 3.4). Normetanephrines and metanephrines are the most confirmatory diagnostic assays for pheochromocytoma. If a patient has elevated metanephrines and normetanephrines while on a VMA-restricted diet, there is a greater than 99 percent probability the patient has a pheochromocytoma.

Small tumors are usually associated with the classic intermittent hypertension of pheochromocytoma. The patient may be normotensive between attacks. These tumors are frequently multiple (15 %) but are not prone to be malignant.

LARGE TUMORS

These tumors are found in older individuals (> 40) and frequently weigh 250 g or more. Because of size, the storage capacity of catecholamines by these pheochromocytomas is enormous. The author recalls one 70-year-old female patient whose tumor contained the equivalent of 1000 ampules of Levophed. Although paroxysmal hypertension occurs in individuals with these large tumors, these patients are also prone to develop sustained hypertension (diastolic pressure > 100 torr) between attacks, unlike the younger patients with smaller tumors. Because of tumor mass, there is a large amount of catecholamine metabolizing enzymes present. Thus, a large percentage of catecholamines released are metabolized and inactivated within the tumor parenchyma before reaching the systemic circulation. This is demonstrated by analysis of urinary catecholamines. The ratio of catecholamine metabolites/free catecholamines is higher (97 ± 30) than with small tumors. Malignancy is higher in this group.

PREOPERATIVE ASSESSMENT OF THE PATIENT WITH PHEOCHROMOCYTOMA

It is in the best interest of the patient with pheochromocytoma that he or she be admitted to the hospital several days prior to anticipated surgery. This allows adequate time for meaningful consultations among surgeon, internist, and anesthesiologist; time for laboratory and diagnostic studies; and an opportunity to carefully observe the effects of preoperative therapy.

This period of observation will allow a careful history and physical examination. Emphasis is placed on degree of severity of the hypertension and whether it has resulted in organ decompensation. Target organs are the heart, kidneys, and brain. In addition to a routine search for myocardial decompensation through physical, ECG, and x-ray tests, a stress test may be warranted. History and neurologic examination can determine if there have been strokes.[7] Table 2 summarizes the more pertinent laboratory tests required.

Table 2. Laboratory Tests of Value in Preoperative Assessment of the Patient with Diagnosed Pheochromocytoma.

1. Serum electrolytes
2. Creatinine, creatinine clearance
3. Fasting blood sugar
4. Serial hematocrits
5. Blood volume (if available)
6. Liver transaminases
7. 24-hour urinary catecholamine and catecholamine metabolite analysis (VMA, free catecholamines, metanephrine, and normetanephrine)

Localization of the tumor is frequently done by computerized axial tomography and/or contrast angiography. As stated previously, urinary catecholamines are of great value in determining whether the tumor is a pure norepinephrine or mixed norepinephrine-epinephrine secretor. (Pure norepinephrine-secreting tumors produce only normetanephrine with no metanephrine in the urine. Intraoperative and preoperative cardiac arrhythmias are less common in the pure norepinephrine secreting tumors.) Caution must be exercised in interpretation of blood catecholamine contents obtained during angiography. Radiographic contrast media can cause release of catecholamines from the normal adrenal gland, giving false positive values.

The patient should be started with the alpha adrenergic receptor blocker phenoxybenzamine.[3, 5] This is a long-acting, noncompetitive blocker of alpha adrenergic receptors. Doses in the average adult begin at one 10 mg tablet three times a day. Each day the patient's blood pressure is measured in the supine and standing positions. Phenoxybenzamine 10 mg per day is added until development of mild orthostatic hypotension is noted. This is the end point for this therapy, and the dosage should remain at the level required for this effect. Response to phenoxybenzamine, in addition to reducing blood pressure to normotensive levels, will produce the following salutory effects:

1. The patient feels better. Paroxysmal attacks are almost entirely ablated by adequate phenoxybenzamine therapy. Behavior and outlook of the patient improves.
2. Fasting blood glucose falls to normal levels.
3. After 3 to 4 days of treatment with phenoxybenzamine, the

hematocrit may fall, indicating a restoration of plasma volume. This is a good prognostic sign. Anemia may be unmasked at this time and can be treated appropriately with packed red blood cells.

4. Ventricular extrasystoles ordinarily disappear. Phenoxybenzamine is very effective in controlling blood pressure elevations caused by pheochromocytoma, and very ineffective controlling hypertension from other causes.

When these features are noted following phenoxybenzamine therapy, the patient is usually ready for surgery. The last dose of phenoxybenzamine should be given the night before surgery. The use of the beta adrenergic receptor blocker propranolol should be reserved for patients with resting tachycardia (>120/min) and ventricular extrasystoles following adequate phenoxybenzamine therapy. The introduction of phenoxybenzamine caused concern by some surgeons that the rise in blood pressure seen with tumor manipulation, a valuable localizing sign, would be lost. It is blunted only—a rise will still occur, but, of less magnitude than in the nonpretreated patient. Phentolamine has been advocated as a substitute for phenoxybenzamine. The problem with phentolamine is its short duration of pharmacologic activity, which precludes smooth, sustained alpha adrenergic blockade.

ANESTHETIC MANAGEMENT

Preoperative medication is at the discretion of the anesthesiologist. There are no practical pharamacologic contraindications to the use of any of the common sedatives, hypnotics, and anticholinergics. The author has employed morphine, diazepam, pentobarbital, scopolamine, and atropine. A well-sedated patient with little respiratory depression is ideal.

Monitor selection is important. Recommended are:

1. ECG
2. Indwelling radial arterial catheter with oscilloscopic blood pressure recording
3. Urinary catheter to measure hourly output
4. Temperature probe
5. Peripheral nerve stimulator
6. Optional Swan-Ganz catheter predicated on patient's myocardial status

Selection of anesthetic techniques has been the subject of many case reports in the literature.[2,5] Regional anesthesia, spinal or epidural, has its proponents, but is difficult at best and has few pharmacologic advantages. Surgical exploration for pheochromocytoma is extensive and requires manipulations high in the abdomen. Therefore, a T2–3 level must be maintained for hours at times. Spinal anesthesia does not block peripheral alpha and beta adrenergic receptors, negating its value as a technique for sympatholysis. Thus, even with a high spinal level, circulating catecholamines are not blunted in action. Since release of the catecholamines from a pheochromocytoma is autonomous of an intact sympathetic nervous system, spinal anesthesia will not decrease the hypertensive crisis. Although Innovar has been advocated in anesthetic management, several case reports indicate that droperidol may, at times, cause a release of catecholamines from these tumors, producing dramatic and threatening blood pressure elevations. Halothane also has had its advocates. It has the advantage of being a potent sympatholytic drug, but has the practical disadvantage of sensitizing the myocardium to circulating catecholamines. Halothane may provoke severe ventricular arrhythmias during surgery. The author has not employed the anesthetic for several years because of these difficulties. Enflurane is preferred because of the low incidence of catecholamine-anesthetic arrhythmias, and the ability to quickly depress blood pressure to counter surges of catecholamines.

Table 3 summarizes a very acceptable anesthetic management. Prevention of succinylcholine-induced muscle fasciculations is mandatory since these may produce a milking action literally squeezing large quantities of catecholamines into the systemic circulation. During this approach, fluid and blood replacement should be generous. These patients are now alpha adernergic receptor blocked with phenoxybenzamine and have resultant increased capacitance volume. Thus, they can usually handle a larger volume load than a similar patient without the block. Ringer's lactate and blood constitute ideal replacement fluids, the requirements predicated on blood loss, blood pressure, venous pressure, and urine output. Although increased inspired concentrations of enflurane are ideal for minor blood pressure rises, the rapidly acting alpha receptor blocker phen-

Table 3. Summary of Suggested Anesthetic Technique for Pheochromocytoma Removal.

1. *d*-tubocurarine (.15–3.0 mg) for precurarization to prevent succinylcholine fasciculations
2. Thiopental for induction
3. Enflurane-nitrous oxide by mask until surgical levels of anesthesia reached
4. Succinylcholine to facilitate endotracheal tube insertion
5. Maintenance of anesthesia with enflurane-nitrous oxide; increase concentration to reduce blood pressure as necessary
6. Skeletal muscle relaxation obtained by *d*-tubocurarine if necessary

tolamine can be used to advantage for more serious increases. It is customarily mixed 10 mg phentolamine/100 ml D5W administered as a drip. Phentolamine lasts approximately 20 minutes. Tachycardia will be observed as phentolamine depresses blood pressure. Nitroprusside can also be employed for this purpose, but phentolamine has two advantages: it blocks alpha adrenergic receptors directly, and no toxicity has been noted following its use. Propranolol may be used in doses of 0.25 to 0.5 mg intravenously to control cardiac rates greater than 120/min. The author has only rarely needed to employ this beta adrenergic blocker intraoperatively.

After the surgeon has clamped the venous outflow of the pheochromocytoma, a rather dramatic fall in blood pressure can be expected. As stated earlier, termination of action of the catecholamines is via neuronal uptake, a process requiring only a few minutes. Proper therapy at this time is volume replacement, blood, and Ringer's lactate. A brief intermittent drip of a directly acting sympathomimetric amine, such as phenylephrine, may be used until volume is restored, but its continued use is usually unwarranted and is frequently dangerous. The drug tends to mask the underlying problem, hypovolemia. Even alpha adrenergically blocked patients have fairly normal blood pressures in the supine position. If no great fall in blood pressure occurs following tumor removal, the anesthesiologist can entertain a high degree of suspicion that another, or multiple tumors exist. At times an intravenous provocative histamine test may be necessary at the time of surgery.

SUMMARY

Anesthetic management of pheochromocytoma should be based on very reliable pharmacologic principles. The aura and mystique surrounding management of this endocrinopathy is not justified. Patient care for this problem is strengthened by increased knowledge of the pathophysiology involved, and anesthesia is rather straightforward and intellectually satisfying.

REFERENCES

1. Brunjes, S., John, V. J., Jr., and Crane, M. A.: *Pheochromocytoma: postoperative shock and blood volume.* N. Engl. J. Med. 262:393, 1960.
2. Cooperman, L. H., Engelman, K., and Mann, P. E. G.: *Anesthetic management of pheochromocytoma employing halothane and beta adrenergic blockade: a report of 14 cases.* Anesthesiology 28:575, 1967.
3. Crago, R. M., Eckholdt, J. W., and Wiswell, J. G.: *Pheochromocytoma: treatment with alpha and beta adrenergic drugs.* J.A.M.A. 202:870, 1970.
4. Crout, J. R.: *Pheochromocytoma.* Pharmacol. Rev. 18:651, 1966.
5. Crout, J. R., and Brown, B. R., Jr.: *Anesthetic management of pheochromocytoma: the value of phenoxybenzamine and methoxyflurane.* Anesthesiology 30:25, 1969.
6. Crout, J. R., Pisano, J. J., and Sjoerdsma, A.: *Urinary excretion of catecholamines and their metabolites in pheochromocytoma.* Am. Heart J. 61:375, 1961.
7. Rosenberg, J. C., and Varco, R. L.: *Physiologic and pharmacologic considerations in the management of pheochromocytoma.* Surg. Clin. North Am. 47:453, 1967.
8. Sjoerdsma, A., Engelman, K., Waldman, T., et al.: *Pheochromocytoma: current concepts of diagnosis and treatment.* Am. Intern. Med. 75:1302, 1966.

INDEX